IN A WORLD OF DEADLY VIRUSES,
IGNORANCE CAN BE FATAL.

EVERYONE SHOULD BE ASKING:

- How do you avoid contracting hepatitis altogether?
- Which strains can be cured and which are chronic?
- Can you get hepatitis from eating strawberries or shellfish?
- How dangerous are eating utensils and public bathrooms?
- Which vaccinations should children be given?
- What do you do if you or someone you know has the disease?

Answering these and many more questions with information from the most recent viral research, this book offers the complete facts on this escalating epidemic . . .

Hepatitis A to G

HEPATITIS
A to G

THE FACTS YOU NEED TO KNOW
ABOUT ALL THE FORMS OF THIS
DANGEROUS DISEASE

Alan Berkman, M.D.

AND

Nicholas Bakalar

WARNER BOOKS

A Time Warner Company

WARNER BOOKS EDITION

Cover design by Elaine Groh
Book design by Stanley S. Drate/Folio Graphics Co. Inc.

Warner Books, Inc.
1271 Avenue of the Americas
New York, NY 10020

Visit our Web site at
www.twbookmark.com

 A Time Warner Company

Printed in the United States of America

First Printing: July 2000

10 9 8 7 6 5 4 3 2 1

To the patients
who have shared their stories
and lives with us.

Contents

Acknowledgments

The authors would like to acknowledge the generous help of Milton Wainberg, M.D., Isela Puello, and Francine Cournos, M.D., in the preparation of this book. Our agent Alexander Hoyt, who combines the attributes of an astute businessman with those of a gentleman and a scholar, was instrumental in getting this project off the ground. Diana Baroni, whose idea this book was, is a young editor who does her editing the old-fashioned way: with a sharp pencil and a blunt professional attitude. To her, our profound respect and our heartfelt thanks.

A Note on Terminology

The word "hepatitis" means inflammation of the liver (just as "appendicitis" means inflammation of the appendix or "rhinitis" means inflammation of the tissues of the nasal passages). The liver can be inflamed for various reasons—among others, excessive alcohol consumption, the ingestion of poisonous chemicals or certain medications, and infection. The word "hepatitis" by itself says nothing about what the cause of the inflammation is.

At the same time, "hepatitis" is most often used by doctors and laymen alike to refer to the diseases caused by certain viruses called hepatitis viruses. If a doctor says, "You have hepatitis," she means that you have a viral disease caused by a virus that attacks the liver, and not necessarily that you have an inflamed liver. When we use the word "hepatitis" in this book, we mean the viral disease, and not, except when we specifically say so, the phenomenon of liver inflammation.

1

Hepatitis A to G
AN INTRODUCTION

On your right side, just above your intestines in front of your kidneys and under your rib cage beneath your lungs, lies the most complex organ in your body: your liver. In most adults, it weighs around three pounds, making it by a considerable margin your largest internal organ. Blood is constantly flowing through this organ—in fact, all the blood in your body flows through it to process useful nutrients and get rid of toxins.

Any irritation of the liver, anything that makes it inflamed, is called hepatitis. But the term is most commonly used to describe a group of infectious diseases caused by a handful of different viruses that attack the liver. These viruses, and their effect on the liver, are the subject of this book. There are vaccines for some of these viruses, but not for all. Some of the diseases they cause are chronic, some come and go like a very bad case of the flu, and some are deadly. Six different kinds of hepatitis, A, B, C, D, E, and G, have now been discovered. Each of these is caused by a different virus. Five of the types cause disease; one, hepatitis G, lives in the blood without causing any apparent illness.

Hepatitis is very common. One hundred and twenty-five thousand new cases of hepatitis A occur every year. In the U.S., five thousand people a year die from hepatitis B. Hepatitis C is the main reason for liver transplantation in the United States—more people get new livers because of hepatitis C infection than because of alcoholism—and more than 240 million people are infected worldwide. Hepatitis E is extremely rare in the United States, but is widespread in other parts of the world where inadequate sanitation allows it to flourish.

Hepatitis A is a nasty disease that can be prevented by a simple and nearly painless vaccination. Hepatitis B, too, can be prevented by a vaccine. But if you contract hepatitis B, you can get a chronic form of it that will be with you for the rest of your life. Hepatitis C is a chronic and sometimes deadly disease with no vaccine, no cure, and a treatment that is effective in only a limited number of cases. A coinfection of hepatitis D with hepatitis B can make the disease much worse. Travelers to endemic areas must be aware of the risks of hepatitis E. In other words, hepatitis is of immediate concern to your health and that of your family. This book is intended to equip you with the knowledge you need to diminish your risk.

The Liver: What It Does, How It Works

The liver does much more than purify the blood and process nutrients. Its healthy functioning is essential to other bodily systems—the blood, bile, lymph, and immune systems—and it also performs more than five hundred chemical functions that make your body work properly, including the following:

- Manufacturing proteins
- Storing certain vitamins, iron and other minerals, and sugars
- Regulating the transport of fat stores and controlling the production and excretion of cholesterol
- Regulating blood clotting
- Producing bile essential to the proper digestion of fats
- Purifying the blood by neutralizing and destroying poisonous substances
- Metabolizing alcohol and other drugs
- Maintaining hormone balance
- Forming blood before birth
- Protecting the body from infection by producing immune factors and removing bacteria from the bloodstream
- Regenerating its own damaged tissue

In short, if your liver is functioning poorly, so is almost everything else in your body. If the liver fails, other organs begin to fail as well. The kidneys, colon, bile duct, lungs, and mucous membranes become poisoned. Rashes, eczema, aches and pains, and organ failures may occur. And finally, the risk of liver cancer increases. So any organism that attacks the liver can cause serious problems everywhere. And that is what, among other things, the hepatitis virus does.

Hepatitis: Inflammation of the Liver

The diagnosis of hepatitis—or at least the recognition of its symptoms—is almost as old as the history of medicine. Hippocrates described epidemic jaundice in the fifth century B.C., and what he was seeing was almost certainly a form of the hepatitis virus (though perhaps not a form we know today). The first recorded cases of hepatitis B (which used to be called serum hepatitis) probably were those following the administration of a smallpox vaccine to German shipyard workers in 1883, and the disease was observed repeatedly during the early and middle parts of the twentieth century following the use of contaminated needles and syringes.

The effect of the various hepatitis viruses on the liver—like the effect of alcohol and other toxins—is to scar it. The initial inflammation caused by the virus induces the body's immune system to fight it with immune cells called lymphocytes. But the lymphocytes, while attacking the virus, also harm the liver. Eventually the liver becomes scarred—this is called fibrosis—and when the scarring is severe enough, it begins to hamper blood flow. This is called cirrhosis, and at this stage blood backs up into other organs and the essential functions the liver performs become more and more difficult, and finally impossible, to accomplish.

As we said above, there are now six different species of hepatitis virus known to infect the blood (and some others that might). These are not really strains of the same virus—they're all different organisms that happen to attack the liver and cause similar symptoms. We include much more detail about their natural histories and effect on humans later in this book, but here's a quick review of the facts about them.

Hepatitis A

In March 1997 hepatitis A (also known as HAV) made the news when 153 cases were reported in Calhoun County, Michigan, and the outbreak was traced to crates of frozen strawberries imported from Mexico. But while foodborne outbreaks like this are serious and must be controlled, they are relatively uncommon. Usually hepatitis A is transmitted by oral contact with the feces of infected people. This can happen in various ways—for example, in nursery schools and day care centers, through contact with infected water in swimming pools, or by eating shellfish that grew in water contaminated with sewage. Hepatitis A can also be transmitted by infected blood, but this is very rare.

Symptoms

Often people who contract hepatitis A have no symptoms at all, and the only way you can tell if they have (or at one time had) the disease is by testing their blood for antibodies to the virus. When there are symptoms, older people usually suffer more than younger people: fever, loss of appetite, nausea, stomachaches, dark urine, and jaundice (yellow skin and eyes) are common. Of course, you can have symptoms very much like these without having hepatitis A—the only way to tell if you have it is with a blood test. The unpleasant symptoms usually last less than two months, but they can persist for as long as six months. The incubation period for the virus is about one month—that is, you can be infected with the virus for about a month, and only then begin to have symptoms.

How Do You Catch It?

HAV is not spread by casual contact in the office, school, or factory. But it is spread by contact within families and by sexual contact. In the great majority of cases, people recover from hepatitis A infection, and, since infection confers immunity, never have to worry about it again. In some cases, however, known as "fulminant hepatitis," the case-fatality rate can be as high as 50 percent despite modern medical interventions such as liver transplantation. About a hundred people a year die from this kind of HAV, usually older people, and often with a preexisting chronic liver disease. If a person is infected with chronic hepatitis C, then hepatitis A infection is a very serious disease with a high fatality rate.

Hepatitis A epidemics are cyclic, occurring about once every ten to fifteen years. The last big epidemic was in 1989. But there is always a large number of people infected—an estimated 125,000 new cases per year.

People most at risk for getting HAV in the United States are children in day care centers and nursery schools and household members of infected people. In the U.S., HAV is largely a pediatric disease—more than 30 percent of reported cases occur in children under fifteen years old, and since most children infected before age five do not have symptoms and are therefore not reported, the actual percentage of cases in children is probably much higher.

Vaccination for Hepatitis A

There is no cure for hepatitis A, but there is a vaccine, and there is a substance—immune globulin—that can be given after infection to prevent, or at least ameliorate, symptoms. Certain groups of people should routinely get the vaccine. And there are important warnings for travelers that must be heeded: intermediate and high rates of HAV cover most of the globe, and travelers to these areas should be vaccinated. Children under two years old cannot be vaccinated. Chapter 2 gives the details. Interestingly, certain people you might think ought to be vaccinated—sewage workers, food service workers, health care workers, and day care attendees—should in fact not be routinely vaccinated.

Hepatitis B

Hepatitis B (HBV) can be a more serious disease than HAV. Unlike HAV, it has both an acute and a chronic form. The incubation period for HBV is between 45 and 180 days—that's how long you can have the infection before you see any symptoms—and the onset of acute disease develops gradually. Doctors call this an "insidious" onset. Not all people who are infected with the virus develop symptoms, and most who do get sick will recover and have immunity from then on. But a large number continue to have chronic infection. Every year in the United States there are about 200,000 new cases of HBV. Eleven thousand of these people get so sick they have to be hospitalized, and 20,000 remain chronically infected. There are now approximately 1.25 million Americans with chronic HBV, and about 5,000 people die each year from the liver disease and liver cancer caused by HBV.

This is a disease of young adults—people between twenty and thirty-nine years of age have the highest rates of infection. Children's rates are relatively low in the United States (and often concentrated in communities of immigrants from countries where rates are high), although rates among kids are higher than the number of reported cases might suggest because asymptomatic cases are common and not noticed. But the disease in young children is very dangerous because 80 to 90 percent of infants infected during the first year of life, and about half of children infected between the ages of one and four, develop chronic HBV infection. HBV can be passed on by infected mothers to their children during childbirth—about a quarter of all chronic HBV infections are acquired in this way.

Symptoms

The symptoms of acute HBV infection are very unpleasant: loss of appetite, tiredness, pain in muscles and joints, stomachaches, diarrhea and vomiting, jaundice. The chronic disease is even worse: it damages the liver in ways that can cause liver cancer and death.

A blood test can determine whether a person has the acute or chronic form of the disease. Recovery from the acute disease generally confers immunity. Sometimes the acute disease becomes chronic—this, too, can be determined by testing the blood.

How Do You Catch It?

HBV is a bloodborne and sexually transmitted disease. The virus is present in the highest concentrations in blood and blood fluids, and in lesser concentrations in semen, vaginal fluid, and saliva. Blood exposure and sexual contact are quite efficient modes of transmission. Although it doesn't happen often, tattooing, ear piercing, acupuncture, and accidental needlesticks can be routes of bloodborne transmission. The cause of perinatal transmission is most often contact of the infant's mucous membranes with maternal blood during delivery. The Centers for Disease Control in Atlanta has concluded that about 50 percent of cases have a sexual risk factor. Men who have sex with men are at particular risk. In fact, the original hepatitis B vaccine trials were carried out among gay men at high risk. Fifteen percent of cases have a drug use risk factor, 4 percent have other risk factors (household contact, health care employment), and 31 percent have no identifiable risk factor.

Vaccination

There is a highly effective and very safe vaccine for HBV, and the current standard is that everyone under eighteen, and those in certain risk groups over eighteen, should be vaccinated (see chapter 3 for the details). The aim of this vaccination policy is the total elimination of HBV virus transmission in the United States, and this is now within reach.

Hepatitis C

This is the nastiest hepatitis variety of all. About 85 percent of people who are infected by this virus never get rid of it. Chronic liver disease afflicts about 70 percent of people who are infected with hepatitis C (HCV), and this can lead to liver cancer and death. Some studies suggest that 40 percent of all liver disease in the United States can be attributed to HCV infection, making it as important a contributor as alcohol abuse. Between 8,000 and 10,000 people a year die from the effects of HCV infection. We can put it this way: of 100 people who get infected with HCV, about 85 will be chronically infected, about 70 will develop chronic liver disease, about 15 will develop cirrhosis over a period of twenty to thirty years, and about 5 will die of cirrhosis or liver cancer. A small percentage of people infected develop "extrahepatic" conditions—that is, conditions that afflict other parts of the body besides the liver.

There are several blood tests, some available only in research projects, that will determine if you have HCV, and chapter 4 explains what the tests involve and what they reveal. A person can be infected for five to six weeks before the currently licensed test reveals antibodies to HCV—though the person may still have no symptoms. Although a small number of HCV cases turn out not to be chronic, there is no test to distinguish acute from chronic disease as there is for HBV.

Symptoms

If symptoms of HCV do appear, they usually take about six to seven weeks after the initial infection, but only about 30 to 40 percent of people infected develop any acute symptoms at all. About a quarter of those who develop symptoms have jaundice. The real problems come later, during the period of chronic infection, when liver disease can develop. Until recently it was believed that most people infected with HCV went on to develop liver disease, but this was probably a mistaken impression left by the fact that only people with symptoms are likely to be diagnosed and treated. In fact, people can be infected for many years without symptoms of any kind.

Treatment

While there is no vaccine for HCV, there is a treatment: antiviral drugs such as interferon are approved for the treatment of chronic HCV. But unfortunately, interferon usually doesn't work: only 15 to 20 percent of people get better on it. When you combine interferon with ribavirin, another antiviral drug, the cure rate goes up to between 30 and 50 percent. Ribavirin used alone is not effective at all. Interferon therapy has many unpleasant, and some dangerous, side effects. Most people who take the drug get flulike symptoms (fever, chills, a fast heart rate, and muscle and joint aching). In time, other side effects may include tiredness, hair loss, low blood count, moodiness, confusion, and depression. Severe side effects (if you don't consider these severe enough) occur in about 2 percent of people on interferon: thyroid disease, depression with suicidal thoughts, seizures, acute heart or kidney failure, eye and lung problems, hearing loss, and blood infection. About 15 percent of people who start interferon treatment can't continue because of these problems. Adding ribavirin makes the treatment more effective, but risks causing serious anemia. Pregnant women cannot use interferon.

There is a further important risk to consider for women of childbearing age: ribavirin can cause severe birth defects. You must use two forms of contraception if you are taking ribavirin.

How Is HCV Transmitted, and Who Is Most Likely to Get It?

If there is any good news about HCV, it is that it isn't easy to get. It is almost exclusively transmitted in infected blood. You can't get it by breast-feeding, sneezing, hugging, coughing, from sharing eating utensils, from food or water, or by casual contact with an infected person.

Still, that leaves quite a few ways in which you *can* contract it. You can get it by injecting drugs—even if you injected only once years ago. You can get it if you were treated with a blood product made before 1987 (clotting factor, for example), or from an infected blood transfusion or a transplanted organ from an infected person. You can get it if you have been on long-term kidney dialysis, from accidental needlesticks if you are a health care worker, from your mother if she had it when you were born, or from sharing items, such as razor blades and toothbrushes, that have infected blood on them. In contrast to HIV and HBV, you are very unlikely to get HCV from sexual contact. But it is possible, most commonly through anal sex. Still, there are many HCV-positive people who do not appear to belong to any of these risk groups.

Although it may be surprising considering all the talk about HCV, there has actually been a decline in infection rates in recent years. This is probably due to some of the behavioral changes that have followed from the HIV epidemic: injection drug users observe safer practices, blood is screened more efficiently, changes in organ donor selection practices have been put into effect, and, since the early 1990s, all donated blood has been screened for HCV. Transmission by sexual, household, and occupational exposure, on the other hand, has remained about the same over time.

Hepatitis D

Hepatitis D (HDV) is sometimes called the delta virus. It can't replicate, or reproduce, without the presence of HBV, which it needs to make the envelope of protein that encapsulates the HDV genome. It coexists with HBV in two ways: as a coinfection (occurring at the same time), or as a superinfection (occurring after hepatitis B infection is already established). A person with an HBV-HDV coinfection may have more severe acute disease and a higher risk of fulminant hepatitis compared with those infected with HBV alone. Yet chronic infection appears to occur less frequently in those with HBV-HDV than in those with HBV alone. People with HBV who then acquire HDV as a superinfection usually become chronically infected—70 to 80 percent of those with HDV superinfection develop chronic liver diseases, compared with 15 to 30 percent of those with HBV infection alone.

Symptoms and Transmission

The symptoms and transmission of HDV are the same as for HBV—it is carried in infected blood and other bodily fluids, and can be transmitted by sexual contact. Sexual transmission is less efficient than for HBV, and perinatal transmission of HDV is rare.

Treatment

Since HDV can only exist in the presence of HBV, the same preventive measures that apply to HBV also apply to HDV. The vaccine prevents both infections, and both can be treated prophylactically with immune globulin after infection. However, there is no way to prevent an HDV superinfection of a person already afflicted with chronic HBV infection.

Hepatitis E

Hepatitis E (HEV) is the enterically transmitted (that is, it is transmitted, like hepatitis A, by oral-fecal contact) non-A, non-B virus. HEV has an incubation period that ranges from two weeks to two months. The signs and symptoms are similar to other kinds of hepatitis: abdominal pain, jaundice, fever, nausea, vomiting, and so on. Diarrhea and various rashes are less common symptoms. The disease is transmitted by contact with the fecal matter of infected people, and is most common in regions with poor sanitation facilities. It is possible that there is a nonhuman carrier of the disease that serves as a reservoir between outbreaks in endemic areas. Unlike HAV, hepatitis E is rarely transmitted person-to-person. Instead, in-

Six kinds of hepatitis: Transmission, symptoms, and treatment

	Hepatitis A	Hepatitis B	Hepatitis C	Hepatitis D	Hepatitis E	Hepatitis G
How it is spread	Through contact with food (uncommonly) or fecal material (usually) that contains the virus.	Exposure to infected blood or blood products, unprotected sex with an infected person, travel to places with high rates of infection. Infected mothers may infect newborns.	Contact with infected blood, including through contaminated needles or sharing razors or toothbrushes with an infected person.	Contact with infected blood, but infection requires the presence of hepatitis B.	Contaminated water or food, particularly in developing countries.	Contact with infected blood.

Symptoms	Fatigue, nausea, vomiting, abdominal pain, dark urine, and jaundice. Tests for liver enzymes may be elevated.	Appetite loss, vomiting, nausea, fever, fatigue, abdominal pain, jaundice. Some people don't have any symptoms.	Most people have none, at least at first. Some have symptoms similar to other forms of hepatitis. Tests for liver enzymes may be elevated.	Same as hepatitis B, but it often makes the symptoms of hepatitis B even more severe.	Abdominal pain, fever, nausea, vomiting, dark urine, jaundice.	Asymptomatic.
Treatment	Bed rest. Can last from three weeks to as long as six months. Immune globulin is used for people already exposed, but there is a vaccine that is highly effective.	Interferon. There is a vaccine that provides immunity and is now recommended for newborns and everyone up to age 18.	Interferon and ribavirin. There is no preventive vaccine.	Interferon to treat hepatitis B.	Bed rest. No drugs or vaccines are available.	None needed.

fected drinking water is the usual route. There have been no documented outbreaks of HEV in the United States, but nevertheless there is a small number of healthy people with antibodies to the disease in their blood. Where this infection comes from, no one knows. There is no vaccine or prophylactic treatment for HEV infection.

Hepatitis G

This is the most recently discovered hepatitis virus, first isolated in a blood sample of a Chicago surgeon. It looks a lot like HCV—that is, it shares about 85 percent of its genetic sequence with that virus. But so far, it doesn't seem to be infectious or to cause illness. In fact, the Chicago surgeon in question is still operating. There are between 900 and 2,000 cases of hepatitis G infection each year in the United States. Chronic infection develops in most infected people, but chronic disease is rare or may not occur at all. Hepatitis G is bloodborne, but there have been no infections found in transfusion recipients since 1991. It can occur as a coinfection with hepatitis C.

2

Hepatitis A

THE VIRUS AT HOME AND AROUND THE WORLD

If you get hepatitis, it will probably be hepatitis A (HAV), the most common form of the disease. HAV used to be called infectious hepatitis, to distinguish it from hepatitis B, which was called serum hepatitis. Of course, this old name was misleading, since both forms of the disease are infectious. But they are transmitted in somewhat different ways.

The hepatitis A virus lives only in humans. Experimental animals can become infected with it, but no other animal except humans gets it naturally. Like other forms of the hepatitis virus, HAV is very stable—it can stay around for months at room temperature and then still infect someone who comes in contact with it. High temperatures (above 185°F) will kill it in a minute or less, and so will formalin and chlorine. Disinfecting surfaces with a 1:100 solution of household bleach in tap water will inactivate HAV.

HAV is enterically transmitted, which is the medical way of saying that you get it by eating it ("enteric" means pertaining to the intestines). While HAV can be transmitted through contaminated blood, this form of transmission is rare. The most common way to get HAV is through infected fecal matter that comes in contact with the mouth. The virus is also transmitted within households and by sexual contact, and through contaminated food. One way the disease can be transmitted is by contact with the diapers of an infected child—since kids under six often have the disease without showing any symptoms, you wouldn't ordinarily know that a child has it. There have been no cases of transmission by saliva, and waterborne outbreaks, while they do occur, are rare. Shellfish eaten raw from contaminated waters can be a source of the virus, and food eaten uncooked that has been washed in contaminated water can also be a route of transmission. Since the virus will not survive high temperatures, cooking food will eliminate any danger of contracting the illness, even if the food was contaminated.

What the Disease Looks Like

Virologists classify HAV as a picornavirus (viruses have species just like other animals and plants). The virus invades your body and lives there without causing any infection for about a month. After that amount of time, it can start to make you sick. But it doesn't always: some people have HAV and never experience any symptoms at all.

When you get HAV, the symptoms are very much like those of other forms of hepatitis—there is a sudden onset of fever, malaise, nausea, vomiting, abdominal pain, dark urine, and jaundice. By the time symptoms appear, the virus has been in your body for between two weeks and

two months—that's known as its "incubation period."
The disease can be persistent, lasting up to two months
in many cases, and in roughly 10 percent of cases going
on for up to six months. The hepatitis A virus replicates
in the liver and disturbs the way it functions. That's why
you get dark urine and jaundice—the functions of the
liver that normally prevent this are being interfered with.

As we noted above, not everyone who is infected
with HAV gets the symptoms of the disease. The older
you are, the more likely you are to have them. Among
children under six, about three-quarters of infections
have no symptoms at all. However, among older children
and adults the picture is reversed: about three-quarters do
have symptoms of one kind or another.

Usually a case of hepatitis A comes and goes—you
simply get better after a period of time. But about a hundred people a year get a deadly form of the disease called
fulminant hepatitis A, which kills them. This is more
common in people over forty—about 2 percent of cases
in this age group are the fulminant variety. The overall
risk for death from HAV is about 0.3 percent, but among
people over the age of fifty the death rate goes up to 1.8
percent. People who have chronic liver disease are also
at considerably higher risk for death.

Even in cases where people recover quickly, the disease can be agonizing. Many are hospitalized and out of
work for a month or more. Since there is no treatment for
HAV, once you get it you just have to try to make yourself
as comfortable as possible and let the illness run its
course. But once it goes away, you're immune. There's
no such thing as chronic hepatitis A infection.

The only way to definitively diagnose HAV is through
a laboratory blood test. The test detects the presence of
an antibody called IgM anti-HAV. If you have this, you've

got the virus. This antibody usually disappears within six months after the onset of symptoms, but after that another antibody, IgG anti-HAV, is still present, and remains in your blood for the rest of your life—and a good thing, too, because this is the antibody that confers lifelong immunity to the disease.

Sicker Than She'd Ever Been

Cindy looked acutely ill. I had seen her for minor health problems some time ago, and I remembered her as an energetic and intelligent young woman. Now, as I approached her in the waiting room, she looked sallow, with her shoulders bent inward and her arms wrapped protectively around herself. I touched her shoulder and asked her to come into my office.

As soon as we were seated looking at each other, I could see that the sclerae (whites) of her eyes were a muddy yellow. I asked her to tell me what had happened.

"I was doing fine until about a few days ago. I felt like I was coming down with the worst flu ever—my entire body hurt, I felt feverish, my stomach hurt, and I was nauseated. I even began to vomit and have diarrhea. Then my urine became dark, I guess because I'm so dehydrated. I've never felt like this."

I asked her if she had noticed any change in her bowel movements, and she said that they were chalky white. Finally, I asked if she had noted the color of her eyes, and she hesitatingly admitted that she had.

While doing her physical exam, I gently palpated her abdomen and felt the solid edge of the liver about two inches below her right ribs. I positioned my fingers along the edge and asked her to first blow out and then take a deep breath in; this caused her liver to lift and move along my fingers. She winced as my hands touched the acutely inflamed organ.

When we were seated again, I explained that she had acute hepatitis, although I couldn't be sure what the cause was until I did some tests. I explained that there was a variety of causes, including viruses, alcohol, some medications, and chemicals. She said that she never drank, took no medications except occasional Tylenol, and had no exposure to chemicals that she was aware of. I asked her what her current job was and she told me she had been working at a day care center for the past year. The children she cared for were as young as eighteen months.

I asked her if any of the children had been sick, but she said some of them were always sick with one virus or another. I was sure she was right—and I suspected that one of the viruses was hepatitis A. I asked her if any of the people she worked with had been sick recently, but none were that she knew of. I told her to stay home from work until we got the test results back, and to be very careful to wash her hands thoroughly every time she used the bathroom. I explained that if she did have hepatitis A, she could accidentally transmit it to others. She said she lived by herself and was not currently in an intimate relationship. I gave her a prescription for something to help with the vomiting, and reminded her to stay away from alcohol and from Tylenol. (In large doses, Tylenol can be extremely poisonous to the liver.) She said friends would visit regularly and check on her, and I told her to call me if she felt worse.

She didn't need to call during the next week and came back for her test results accompanied by a friend. She said she was feeling a bit better, and she looked less ill. I explained that her liver function tests had confirmed the acute hepatitis: her AST and ALT were more than ten times normal, and her bilirubin, the substance that gave her eyes and skin that yellowish appearance, was moderately high at 8.7. Her liver serologies showed that she had acute hepatitis A (her IgM was positive and her IgG negative), and she had never been infected with either hepatitis B or C.

I assured her that she would continue to improve and should be feeling almost normal in a couple of weeks; it was a rare case of hepatitis A that lasted longer than four to six weeks. Assuming she continued to feel better, I wanted her to return in three weeks to do her liver function tests again, and we would talk about her getting hepatitis B vaccine sometime in the future. There was one other thing: it was likely that she got the hepatitis virus from one of the children, and I was going to let the Health Department know about it so they could determine if any other cases involved the same day care center. If they suspected an epidemic, they could offer vaccine to the staff and to children older than two years.

Cindy was pretty much back to normal when she returned for the final set of blood tests. She was ready to return to work, and had heard from some of her coworkers that most of them had gotten the first of the two injections of the hepatitis A vaccine. She commented that she had never felt so sick in her life. I assured her that she was now resistant to hepatitis A, and that after her liver totally normalized for a few months, she would start the three-injection hepatitis B vaccine. Hopefully, she would never be that sick again in her life.

As with many illnesses, by the time you have symptoms, you're not particularly infectious anymore. With HAV, the most infectious period occurs one to two weeks *before* the person shows signs of being sick—that's when there's the most HAV virus in the stool, and when a person is most likely to give it to someone else. By the time the person appears jaundiced, the risk decreases considerably, and it becomes minimal a week after that.

Many people think of hepatitis A as "that disease you get from rotten shellfish," but in fact contaminated shellfish or other food accounts for only about 2 or 3 percent of cases in the United States. (By the way, shellfish or other food contaminated with HAV is not necessarily "rotten." The hepatitis A virus has no taste, and food contaminated with it can taste just fine.) Food can be contaminated by a food handler who has HAV—in fact, it was the danger of HAV transmission that made most health departments impose the regulation that requires the "Employees must wash hands" sign in restaurant bathrooms. When foodborne outbreaks do occur, of course, they require intensive public health efforts to control them, and the publicity such efforts receive may be the reason why many people believe that food is a common source of hepatitis A, which it is not.

Some 22 to 26 percent of cases come from sexual contact or household contact with an infected person. Fourteen to 16 percent are among kids in day care and their caretakers. And between 4 and 6 percent of cases come from people who caught HAV in another country. That takes care of half the cases. The other half? No one knows where they caught the virus, but the guess is they got it from someone they didn't know was infected. This makes sense—as we know, people are most infectious before they have symptoms, and many people go through the course of the disease and become infectious without ever having any symptoms at all.

There are certain groups of people who are considered at higher risk than others: international travelers, men who have sex with men, and drug users. Some groups that you'd think might be at higher risk are not: health care workers, workers exposed to sewage, and food handlers, for example, are at no higher risk than anyone else. Even though there have been reported outbreaks in neonatal intensive care units and in association with adult fecal incontinence, hospital workers are not a risk group. Schools are not common sites for HAV transmission (HAV among schoolchildren usually just reflects the rates in the rest of the community), and there is only one occupational group known to be at increased risk for HAV: people who work with nonhuman primates.

People who have chronic liver disease are not at increased risk for getting HAV, but if they do get it they have a greater chance of contracting the deadly fulminant variety.

The Epidemiology of HAV

Hepatitis A is always around—an average of 27,000 cases a year are reported to the Centers for Disease Control—but every ten years or so there is an epidemic. The most recent one occurred in 1989. The CDC first began taking reports on the disease in 1966, and the largest epidemic since that time was in 1971, when 59,606 cases were reported. The estimated incidence of the disease, taking into account unreported and asymptomatic (and therefore unnoticed) cases, is between 80,000 and 134,000 cases per year. About one-third of the population of the United States has been infected and is immune.

HAV often occurs in community-wide epidemics that may go on for several years and in which as much as 2 percent of the population per year get infected, mostly adults. These communities include American Indian, Alaskan Native, Pacific Islander, certain Hispanic com-

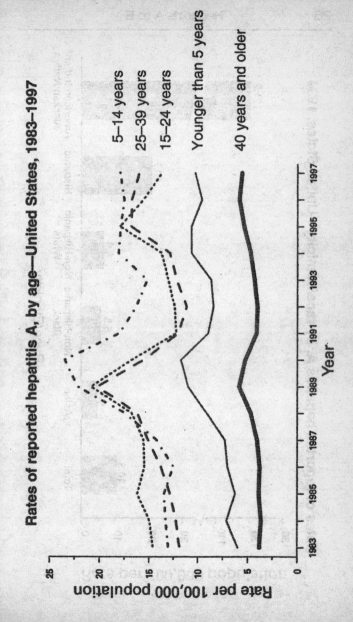

Rates of reported hepatitis A, by age—United States, 1983–1997

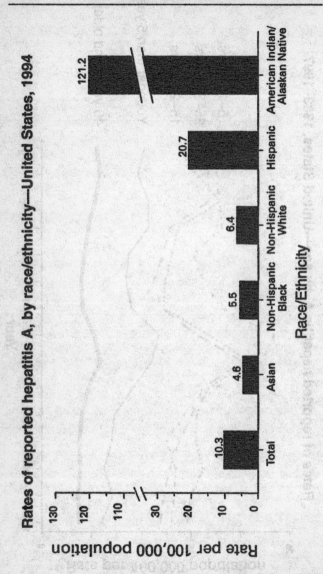

Rates of reported hepatitis A, by race/ethnicity—United States, 1994

munities, and some religious communities. This is probably not a function of genetics, but rather a result of crowded living conditions, poor sanitation, or both. In other communities HAV occurs mainly among children, adolescents, and young adults, again in regularly occurring epidemics, but with lower rates of around 50 to 200 cases per 100,000 population. During these outbreaks, young children who are infected but have no symptoms of disease are a source of infection for their elders. When these outbreaks are treated with postexposure prophylaxis with immune globulin (see below), this slows transmission but doesn't stop the outbreak.

In communities that have high rates of HAV, epidemics typically occur every five to ten years, and they last several years. There are few cases among people older than fifteen. In these communities, about one-third of kids acquire immunity before they are five years old, and almost everyone becomes infected before reaching young adulthood.

In communities that have intermediate rates of HAV, the pattern is a little different. Most of the disease occurs among children, adolescents, and young adults in these places, which are often in large metropolitan areas. Sometimes the disease is concentrated in specific small neighborhoods. During the periodic epidemics in these areas, HAV infection increases among all age groups, not just kids.

So hepatitis A is largely a young person's disease. Almost 30 percent of cases are among people under the age of fifteen, and the highest rates are among kids between five and fourteen. The older you get, the more likely you are to have the HAV antibody (IgG anti-HAV) in your blood. Of Americans over seventy, 75 percent are immune to HAV. The number of people who have the antibody is inversely proportional to their income—in other words, poor people are more likely to have been exposed to the disease than rich people. Mexican Americans (67 percent) have a higher rate of immunity than blacks (37 percent); blacks have a higher rate than whites (29 percent).

In the United States, there is considerable geographic variation in the rate of HAV infections. Western states have higher rates than other parts of the country. The highest rates are in Arizona, Alaska, New Mexico, Oregon, Utah, and Washington, with California, Oklahoma, South Dakota, Idaho, and Nevada not far behind.

In communities that have high rates of HAV epidemics typically occur every few years and may last several years. There is a tendency among people older

Risk Groups

Tourists, military personnel, missionaries, and people who go to work in foreign countries that have intermediate or high levels of HAV endemicity are a group at elevated risk for HAV infection. Staying in urban areas or in luxury hotels won't protect you—viruses don't really care how rich you are—nor will trying to stay away from the water or observing other protective measures. Even if while visiting a foreign country you actually could completely isolate yourself from any contact with the people or culture, you still couldn't protect yourself from HAV (although you would surely ruin your vacation). You will, in one way or another, come in contact with local conditions. You're in this high-risk group if you're in endemic areas no matter what you do or how careful you are. The only sure protection is vaccination.

Recent outbreaks among men who have sex with men have been reported in urban areas in the United States, Canada, and Australia. Rates among this population are several times as high as the rest of the community. When

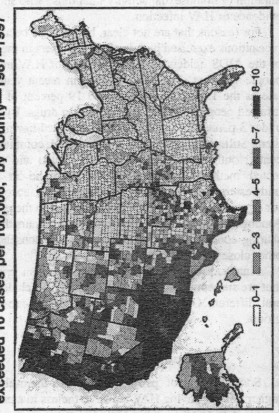

Number of years that reported incidence of hepatitis A exceeded 10 cases per 100,000,* by county—1987–1997

0-1 2-3 4-5 6-7 8-10

*Approximately the national average during 1987–1997.

surveys are done of gay men, those with HAV antibodies (that is, those who have been infected) report more frequent oral-anal contact, more sexual partners, and longer duration of homosexual activity than those who show no evidence of HAV infection.

For reasons that are not clear, but perhaps because of precautions exercised by injection drug users in the wake of the AIDS epidemic, the percentage of HAV-infected people who use drugs has declined in recent years. As late as the 1980s, between 10 and 19 percent of HAV-infected people reported using injection drugs. By 1996, under 3 percent of infected people reported having used them. Still, outbreaks among drug users are common. Recently, outbreaks among users of injected and noninjected methamphetamine have been found in many midwestern and western U.S. communities, accounting for as much as 30 percent of reported cases in these areas. Among drug users, transmission probably occurs through sharing contaminated needles and through household or other close personal contact.

Finally, people who work with nonhuman primates that are susceptible to HAV infection—this includes several different Old and New World species—are a risk group.

Risk among Other Groups

Some groups of people, while not themselves at higher risk for having HAV, are nevertheless in a position to pass it on to others when they do have it.

Being a food service worker, for example, unlike being a traveler in a part of the world with endemic HAV, does not in itself put you at higher risk for HAV, so food service workers are not considered a risk group. Foodborne outbreaks, as we said earlier, are not common in the United States, but they do occur, usually because the food has been prepared by an infected person. So food handlers may pass on HAV, but they are not at increased risk simply because of their occupation—they have the same rates of HAV as everyone else, but they're in a position to pass it on to others.

People with chronic liver disease are another group like this. They don't have higher rates of HAV because they have liver problems, but there is a high prevalence of chronic liver disease among people who died of fulminant hepatitis A. This is because the same kinds of behaviors that harm the liver also put people at risk for multiple infections.

People who work in day care centers, and the kids who attend them, are, like food service workers, in a position to pass on the disease, even though their rates are no higher than those of any other group. Since most kids who have HAV don't have any symptoms, the disease often only becomes apparent when they pass it on to an adult. Kids who don't wash their hands after they use the bathroom, and adults who aren't careful when they handle dirty diapers, are good transmitters of HAV. Outbreaks are rare in day care centers where the kids have to be old enough to be out of diapers to attend. There is no increased prevalence of HAV infection among children and adolescents who previously attended day care centers. Rarely, infection in day care centers is a source of infection in the wider community. Much more commonly, it's the other way around: highly infected communities infect day care centers as they do other places. There is no reason for anyone to avoid putting their kids in day care because of fear of HAV infection.

You might think that people who work in hospitals

would be at higher risk for HAV, but they aren't. This is probably because when you are hospitalized for HAV, it's usually after you have symptoms, and, as we said, after you have symptoms you aren't particularly infectious. There are, however, sporadic outbreaks in hospitals and in institutions for people with developmental disabilities, usually associated with fecal incontinence. Still, a health care worker is no more likely to be infected with HAV than any other worker.

Even though HAV is largely a disease of children, children don't often pass it from one to the other. That's why schools are not usually a source of HAV infection. If there is an outbreak in a school, you should look for a common source of the infection. It probably is *not* coming from other kids.

Finally, in the United States, no work-related cases of HAV transmission have been reported among workers exposed to sewage. There have been waterborne outbreaks of HAV that are not apparently associated with fecal matter in the water, but these are extremely rare.

Reporting on the Epidemic

HAV is a reportable disease—that is, health care workers and hospitals are required by law to report cases of HAV to the health department. The reasons are several. Public health authorities want to monitor the disease incidence in various age groups, determine the characteristics of those infected, discover the source of the infection, identify contacts of infected people to be sure they get postexposure prophylaxis, spot outbreaks as they occur, and determine the effectiveness of the vaccine. Sporadic cases are reported, but not usually investigated. When

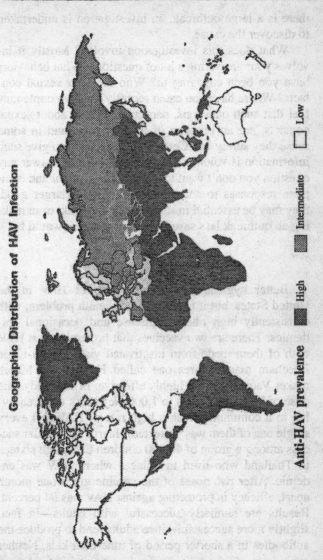

Geographic Distribution of HAV Infection

Anti-HAV prevalence

■ High
▨ Intermediate
□ Low

there is a large outbreak, an investigation is undertaken to discover the cause.

What does this investigation involve? Mostly it involves your answering a lot of questions: What behaviors have you been engaging in? Who are your sexual contacts? Where have you eaten recently? Many people may feel that such questions, particularly those about sexual contacts, are an invasion of their privacy, and in some sense they surely are. Certainly the decision to give such information is voluntary—you don't have to answer any question you don't want to answer. But truthful and complete responses to such questions serve a larger good: they may be essential in stopping an outbreak, or in making an outbreak less severe than it otherwise would be.

The Hepatitis A Vaccine

Better hygiene has reduced rates of HAV in the United States, but it is still a major health problem, with consistently high rates of disease and occasional epidemics. There are two vaccines that protect against HAV, both of them made from inactivated virus. Smith-Kline Beecham manufactures one called Havrix, and Merck makes Vaqta. Both are highly effective. In one study, one dose of Vaqta was given to 1,000 New York children living in a community with a high rate of HAV, and every single one of them was protected. Havrix had similar success among a group of 40,000 children under age sixteen in Thailand who lived in villages where HAV was endemic. After two doses of the vaccine given one month apart, efficacy in protecting against HAV was 94 percent. Results are similarly successful with adults—in fact, slightly more successful, since adults tend to produce the antibodies in a shorter period of time than kids. Neither of these vaccines is approved for infants under two years of age.

How long the protection offered by these vaccines lasts is still an open question, because they've only been used for six or seven years. But there is good reason to believe from observations made so far that the protection from one vaccine series will last as long as twenty years. The need for booster shots will be determined by surveillance studies conducted over time, but currently no booster shots are recommended.

Who Should Get the Vaccine?

The CDC would like to see the incidence of HAV lowered by wider use of the vaccine against it, especially in those populations discussed above where the disease is endemic. Vaccination in those populations would help to eliminate one of the reservoirs of the disease. The most effective way to control hepatitis A would be to incorporate the vaccine into routine childhood vaccination schedules. Unfortunately, the vaccine now available is not suitable for kids under two years old, so this is not now possible.

For now, unlike the vaccination for hepatitis B, the vaccination for hepatitis A is not routinely recommended for everyone. The CDC wants to concentrate instead on certain groups. If you (and anyone else with you who is more than two years old) are traveling to or working in a country where hepatitis A is endemic, however, you should get the vaccine (see below for what to do about infants). This includes most of the world, with the exception of western Europe, North America, Scandinavia, Japan, New Zealand, and Australia. If you get the first dose four weeks before you travel, you will be protected, but you should get the second dose six to twelve months after that.

Routine hepatitis A vaccination of children over the age of two is now recommended in places where the rates of HAV exceed 20 cases per 100,000 population—about twice the national average. This includes many urban areas all over the country, and the following states: Alaska, Arizona, California, Idaho, Nevada, New Mexico, Oklahoma, Oregon, South Dakota, Utah, and Washington. Vaccination may also be considered in communities where the rate is between 10 and 20 cases per 100,000 population. This would add many cities and the following states to the list: Arkansas, Colorado, Missouri, Montana, Texas, and Wyoming.

Men who have sex with men, injection drug users, and people with chronic liver disease or an occupational risk of infection should also get the vaccine. As we will see later in this book, people with hepatitis C should be vaccinated against hepatitis A and hepatitis B.

Hepatitis A Vaccine: Who Should Have It

- People traveling or working in countries with high or intermediate endemicity of HAV
- Children over two years old living in communities with high rates of HAV and periodic epidemics
- Men who have sex with men
- Illicit drug users, both injecting and noninjecting
- All people with hemophilia who receive replacement therapy
- People at occupational risk
- People with chronic liver disease

There isn't any danger in getting the vaccine if you're already immune, but it may be cheaper to screen for immunity than to get unnecessary shots. People who are immune compromised can get the vaccine safely because it is inactivated.

There are no studies of the safety of hepatitis A vaccine for pregnant women, but the theoretical risk to the woman or her developing fetus seems to be very low since the vaccine is produced from inactivated HAV. The risk should be weighed against the risk of HAV infection. You should of course consult with your doctor before deciding to get this or any other vaccine.

The vaccines have few side effects, the most common of which are soreness or tenderness at the injection site. A much smaller number of people report headaches or malaise.

Havrix comes in two different formulations for kids up to age eighteen, and one for adults. (The pediatric formulations vary in amount and dosage schedule—the actual vaccine is the same.) Your doctor will give you the injection in your shoulder, in the manufacturer's recommended doses below. Havrix should be avoided by anyone with a sensitivity to alum or to the preservative 2-phenoxyethanol.

Recommended doses of Havrix® hepatitis A vaccine

Age	Dose (EL.U)*	Volume	No. doses	Schedule
2–18	720	0.5 ml	2	1 to 12 months apart†
Over 18	1,440	1 ml	2	6 to 12 months apart

*ELISA units

†Or 360 EL.U per .5 ml in 3 doses, the second 1 month after the first, the third 6 to 12 months after that.

Vaqta also comes in adult and pediatric formulations, which vary only in the amount of product. It is also administered in the shoulder muscle. Vaqta should be avoided by anyone with an allergy to alum.

Recommended doses of Vaqta® hepatitis A vaccine

Age	Dose (U)*	Volume	No. doses	Schedule
2–17	25	0.5 ml	2	6 to 18 months apart
Over 17	50	1 ml	2	6 months apart

*Units of antigen

Normally you should get the same brand of vaccine for each shot, but if for some reason the same brand isn't available, the other one can be used by your physician. Adults can get the hepatitis A vaccine along with other vaccines without decreasing its effectiveness or increasing adverse events. Studies are under way to determine if this is true with children as well.

The vaccines for hepatitis A and hepatitis B can be given at the same time, although the injections should be at different sites. The CDC has encouraged the development of combination vaccines for more efficient immunization, and in fact there are now combination vaccines for hepatitis A and hepatitis B. As of this writing, they are available only in Europe, and are still being evaluated for use in the United States. It is not currently known when the vaccine will be available in this country.

Vaccination in Outbreaks

The vaccine is highly effective in controlling community outbreaks of hepatitis A. In communities that have high rates of hepatitis A, vaccinating children aged two to sixteen years results in substantial decreases in HAV rates, and if you continue vaccinating you prevent future outbreaks as well. In several Alaskan villages where HAV outbreaks were occurring, vaccination of children and adults quickly resulted in a decrease in the number of new cases. Similar good results were achieved in American Indian communities where outbreaks were beginning—the outbreaks were stopped completely. Even in communities with only mild rates of HAV—Butte County, California, and Memphis, Tennessee, for example—hepatitis A incidence decreased sharply as soon as vaccination programs were implemented.

Immune Globulin: What It Is, and Who Should Get It

In addition to the two vaccines, there is a third protective measure that your doctor may advise you to take. Standard immune globulin (IG; this used to be called gamma globulin) is a concentrated solution of antibodies extracted from human blood plasma, and provides protection against HAV. This form of immunization is not as effective as the vaccines and has only a temporary effect, but it is useful for preventing symptoms after exposure, and can be used in certain other situations, as we will see below. Children under two years, who cannot take the vaccine, can only be immunized with IG. The reason for this is that antibodies an infant acquires from its mother interfere with the effect of the vaccine. Studies are under way now to determine the right dose and timing of vaccinations for infants, but as of this writing the results are not yet available and the hepatitis A vaccine is not licensed for use with infants.

Immune globulin for the prevention of HAV infection is administered in an intramuscular shot. When this is done within two weeks of the exposure, it is more than 85 percent effective in preventing the disease. The earlier you get the immune globulin after exposure to HAV, the more effective it is in preventing it.

IG is prepared from blood plasma. The plasma of many different immune people is pooled, and then, by a process called cold ethanol fractionation, the final product is produced. This plasma has been shown to be very safe in the United States: it has been tested negative for hepatitis B surface antigen, negative for HIV, and negative for the antibody to hepatitis C virus. Moreover, the process of cold ethanol fractionation can itself eliminate and inactivate HIV.

Immune globulin transfers antibodies produced by a group of immune people into the blood of the person getting the intramuscular shot. The levels of antibodies achieved this way are too low to be detected by the regular test for the anti-HAV antigens, but they are enough to provide immunity. The concentration of anti-HAV differs depending on the lot the IG comes from, and, because of decreasing levels of HAV among plasma donors, there has been a decrease in the concentration in recent years. But there is no evidence of a decrease in IG's protective effect.

IG is used for the postexposure management of the disease, so doctors recommend that people should get it if they have had close contact, either sexual or within a household, with a person who has HAV. Staff and children at child care centers where a case of hepatitis A has been found should also be given IG, as should people in certain exposure situations, such as patrons of a food establishment where a staff member has been found to have HAV. People who have been vaccinated at least one month before exposure, even if they have gotten only one of the two doses, usually do not need IG. The correct dose of IG depends on your weight and whether you're getting it before you've been exposed or after.

Recommended doses of IG for hepatitis A preexposure and postexposure prophylaxis

Setting	Duration of Coverage	Dose*
Preexposure	Short-term (1–2 months)	0.02 ml/kg†
	Long-term (3–5 months)	0.06 ml/kg
Postexposure		0.02 ml/kg

*IG is given by intramuscular injection into either the arm or the buttock. Infants less than two years old get it in the thigh muscle.

†Repeated every 5 months if continued exposure to HAV occurs.

If you are traveling to an endemic area in less than four weeks you should get IG, too, and the shot should be repeated if you stay in the area for more than five months. Anyone with an allergy or sensitivity to alum should get IG instead of the vaccines.

IG does not interfere with vaccines for oral polio virus, yellow fever, oral typhoid, cholera, Japanese encephalitis, or rabies, or with the vaccine for hepatitis B. But it can interfere with the action of live, attenuated vaccines like those for measles, mumps, rubella, and varicella. Therefore, these vaccines shouldn't be given until at least three months after the administration of IG. And conversely, unless the benefits of giving IG prophylaxis exceed the benefits of the other vaccinations, you shouldn't have IG for two weeks after a vaccination for measles, mumps, or rubella, and for at least three weeks after a varicella vaccination.

Since infants cannot be given either of the vaccines for hepatitis A, if you are traveling with an infant to a country where hepatitis A is endemic, you should consult with your pediatrician about treating your infant with IG.

For travelers, the dosage of IG takes some figuring—it depends on your body weight and how long you are staying in an endemic area. The table below summarizes the information.

Immune globulin for protection against hepatitis A among travelers

Length of stay	Body weight	Dose volume
Less than 3 months	Less than 50 pounds	0.5 ml
	50 to 100 pounds	1 ml
	Over 100 pounds	2 ml
3 to 5 months	Less than 22 pounds	0.5 ml
	22 to 50 pounds	1 ml
	50 to 100 pounds	2.5 ml
	More than 100 pounds	5 ml

Immune globulin prepared in the United States and administered intramuscularly has few side effects, the most common of which is soreness at the injection site. It has never been shown to transmit infectious agents. Even pregnant women, under their doctor's supervision, have taken IG safely. Of course, getting the hepatitis A vaccine is better protection: protection with IG doesn't last more than about six months, while the vaccine provides protection for at least twenty years, and very likely for a lifetime.

3

Hepatitis B
A RISK YOU CAN ELIMINATE

In the early 1960s, a researcher named Baruch Blumberg was doing research on serum polymorphism—the phenomenon of the body using proteins that differ in structure to achieve the same function (two examples are proteins in milk and in hemoglobin). Such polymorphisms are most often found in isolated and homogeneous populations and one such group is Australian aborigines, so Dr. Blumberg was working with blood samples from this group.

Dr. Blumberg also examined blood from subjects who received multiple transfusions, reasoning that it might contain antibodies to a range of human proteins (if the donor blood had a slightly different protein from that of the recipient, the recipient would form antibodies).

Dr. Blumberg isolated a novel protein from a specimen from an Australian aborigine in 1963 and called it the Australia antigen. Assuming that it was solely a genetic variant, he must have been surprised when he found the "Australian antigen" was present in many of the specimens from multiply transfused patients. By 1968, he and others demonstrated that Australia antigen was specifically associated with patients who had what was then known as serum hepatitis—what we now call hepatitis B. We now know that Australia antigen is actually HBsAg, which is produced in great quantity by patients with active hepatitis. For his work in this area, Dr. Blumberg shared the Nobel Prize in Medicine or Physiology in 1976.

Worldwide, hepatitis B is a significant public health problem. In Southeast Asia, China, and Africa, more than half the population becomes infected with the virus at some time during their lives, and about 8 percent are chronic carriers. In these areas, transmission from mother to child and among young children is common. In North America and western Europe, where the disease is less common, it is usually transmitted from one adult to another. The World Health Organization estimates that 400 million people are now infected, and that the number of new infections will keep increasing until vaccination of infants is a universally established practice.

The hepatitis B virus is very durable. It can remain infectious on environmental surfaces for at least a month if left at room temperature. Most people who get it fight off the infection by themselves, but the HBV antibodies will be present in their blood for the rest of their lives. Because you can be infected with HBV without having any symptoms, many people are surprised when they go to donate blood to learn that at one time in the past they had the virus. One in every twenty Americans will get HBV at some time in their lives.

Acute and Chronic HBV

Sometimes people infected with HBV have what looks like the flu, with symptoms including loss of appetite, nausea and vomiting, fever, and weakness. They may also develop symptoms more directly related to their livers: abdominal pain, dark urine, jaundice. That kind of HBV infection is usually harmless, even if it can be a little unpleasant for a period of time. But about 5 to 10 percent of people who are infected develop chronic HBV. This is a very serious disease, which can lead to chronic liver disease, cirrhosis, liver cancer, and death. In fact, chronic HBV infection is the most common cause of liver cancer worldwide, and liver cancer is the third most common cancer in the world.

So there are two forms of hepatitis B, one acute and the other chronic. The acute disease is very unpleasant, but if you recover from it you are likely to be immune from then on. Unfortunately, sometimes the acute disease progresses to the chronic form. A blood test—it detects an antibody called IgM anti-HBc—can determine if you have the acute form of the disease.

The immune system usually fights off HBV successfully, but the process is a double-edged sword. While the immune response destroys the virus, it also destroys liver cells—in fact it is the immune response, and not the virus itself, that causes the liver inflammation that can lead to serious liver disease.

The acute disease looks like other forms of acute viral hepatitis. Symptoms tend to appear from forty-five days to five and a half months after infection, and adults suffer more symptoms than infants or children, who usually have no symptoms at all. The disease comes on gradually, with loss of appetite, nausea, and vomiting; pain in the upper right side of the abdomen; headache, skin rashes, and muscle and joint pain. This lasts from three to ten days. Then the patient has dark urine about two days before jaundice sets in. During this period, which lasts one to three weeks, the patient has yellowish skin, light or gray stools, and enlargement of the liver and sometimes of the spleen as well. As the disease goes away, the most persistent symptoms are malaise and fatigue, which can last for weeks or months after the other symptoms have disappeared.

Most people recover completely from acute hepatitis B infection, but about 1 to 2 percent develop fulminant hepatitis, which has mortality rates of 63 to 93 percent. In the United States, about 350 to 450 people per year die from this. Despite this ugly statistic, the real problem with HBV is not the acute infection but the chronic infection, which can be even more deadly.

Of the 200,000 new cases of hepatitis B every year, somewhere between 8,400 and 19,000 people get so sick they need to be hospitalized. All told, 1.25 million people in the U.S. have HBV. About 6 to 10 percent of HBV infections become chronic, and more than 5,000 people a year die from the liver disease HBV causes. The irony of all this is that there is a highly effective and very safe vaccine for HBV that could have prevented almost every one of these cases and that has been in use in the United States for more than fifteen years. In fact, the vaccine is so effective that the Centers for Disease Control believes that transmission of the disease could be totally eliminated with an effective vaccination program. This is what the CDC set out to do in 1991, but the program has not yet succeeded.

Mothers and Children

Children can get HBV at birth if their mothers are infected. In fact, the chance that a mother will pass on the infection during childbirth is quite high. These children, if left untreated, do not have a bright future. Ninety percent of them will have chronic infection, and as many as 25 percent will die of chronic liver disease as adults. A large majority of these infections—up to 90 percent, the CDC estimates—would be prevented if infected mothers were identified and their children given hepatitis B vaccine and hepatitis B immune globulin (HBIG) soon after birth. If this procedure is followed, babies can be safe from HBV infection. They can even breast-feed, since the infection is not passed along in breast milk.

The perinatal (the medical term for something that happens during or just after childbirth) transmission of HBV is more common in other countries than in the United States. But each year an estimated 150,000 children are born to women in the U.S. who have immigrated from places where HBV is endemic. These children are at risk. There are also certain American racial or ethnic groups who are at high risk—Alaskan Natives and Pacific Islanders, for example. In fact, if your parents were born in Southeast Asia, Africa, the Amazon basin in South America, the Pacific islands, or the Middle East, you are at higher risk for HBV. In other words, perinatal transmission of the disease is a significant problem, even though most HBV infections in the United States are acquired by adolescents and adults. HBV vaccination has now been instituted as part of the routine vaccination schedules for infants and children. This has been very effective: among Alaskan Natives, for example, routine vaccination, begun in 1982, has decreased the incidence of acute HBV by more than 99 percent. But it has not eliminated it, and children in these groups continue to be at high risk for infection.

Other HBV Risk Groups

The children of HBV-infected mothers are not the only risk group, and in the United States they are not even the largest risk group. Among adolescents and adults, who constitute a much larger part of the infected population, HBV is transmitted in various ways: sexual contact, especially among homosexual men and people with many heterosexual partners; injection drug use; occupational exposure (among health care workers, for example); household contact with someone who has an acute infection or is a chronic carrier of the virus (this can be by some inadvertent contact with blood, such as that left on a razor or toothbrush); and blood or blood product transfusion. And there is still considerable mystery about HBV infection: despite what is known about these routes of transmission, almost one-third of people with HBV do not have any identifiable risk factor at all. Rates of infection differ among various racial groups: prevalence of the infection among blacks is three to four times greater than among whites.

There are no documented cases of hepatitis B being transmitted by a person being breathed on by someone with the illness, catching it from an insect bite, or getting it through contaminated water.

Vaccination programs for these risk groups have not been very effective in reducing transmission. Three doses of the vaccine are required, and it has been difficult to persuade injection drug users, for example, to follow through on all three shots. Sometimes health care providers are not aware of which groups are at high risk, and so do not identify people who should be vaccinated. Screening of blood donations has revealed carriers, but efforts to vaccinate their household members and sexual contacts have met with limited success. Health care workers have had somewhat better luck: vaccination among this group has reduced rates of infection. But none of this has had much effect on the general rates of HBV infection.

By 1997, about 84 percent of children between nineteen and thirty-five months of age had been vaccinated. Although no figures are available for kids aged eleven and twelve years, many states have implemented middle-school entry requirements for hepatitis B vaccination, so coverage will increase among these preteens.

Vaccination for HBV

The CDC now urges that infants receive the hepatitis B vaccine during routine health care visits, and urges the development of combination vaccines that would include, for example, diphtheria, tetanus, and pertussis vaccines along with the vaccine for HBV. (The Food and Drug Administration did in fact recently approve Comvax, a vaccine that combines an HBV vaccine, Recombivax, with a vaccine for *Haemophilus influenzae* type b.) Still, most cases of HBV in the United States are among adolescents and adults, so vaccinating such at-risk populations is essential as well. The Advisory Committee on Immunization Practices now recommends that all unvaccinated children up to nineteen years old should have the vaccination whenever they are seen for routine medical visits.

The CDC expects that these various efforts to achieve universal vaccination will result in a highly immune population in the United States. Still, much work remains to be done among the children of Alaskan Natives, Pacific Islanders, and immigrant groups from countries where HBV is endemic. Also, because most HBV cases occur among adults, these childhood vaccination programs, even if they are carried out perfectly, will not have an effect in lowering incidence for several years. The solution for the adult group is access to vaccination for groups at high risk: health care workers, people who work with the developmentally disabled, hemodialysis patients, homosexually active men, injection drug users, recipients of blood or blood products, household and sexual contacts of HBV carriers, adoptees from countries with high or intermediate levels of HBV endemicity, Alaskan and Pacific island populations, refugees from areas with high rates of HBV, and long-term prison inmates.

Even if you aren't in any of these risk groups, you may need the vaccine anyway because you must be vaccinated at least six months before travel to areas with high rates of HBV infection. Which parts of the world have high rates of HBV infection? All of Africa, China, Korea, Indonesia, and the Philippines; all of the Middle East except Israel; southern and western Pacific islands; Alaska, Greenland, and the most northern parts of Canada; the interior Amazon basin; and parts of the Caribbean, especially Haiti and the Dominican Republic. Rates are moderate in south central and southwest Asia, Israel, Japan, eastern Europe, Spain, Portugal, Italy, and Russia. And rates are low in northern and western Europe, North America, Australia, and New Zealand.

Traveling in any of these parts of the world doesn't mean you'll necessarily be exposed to HBV, but your risk of exposure is increased by the prevalence of HBV carri-

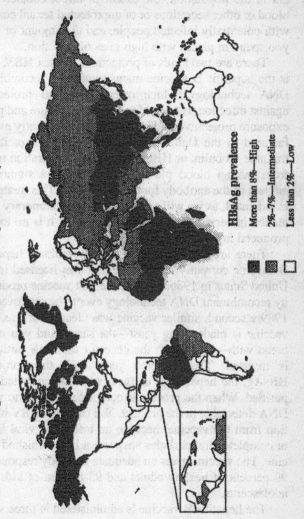

Geographic distribution of hepatitis B prevalence

HBsAg prevalence

- More than 8% — High
- 2%–7% — Intermediate
- Less than 2% — Low

ers in the population, the extent of direct contact with blood or other secretions or of unprotected sexual contact with potentially infected people, and the amount of time you spend in places with high rates of infection.

There are two kinds of protections against HBV. One is the hepatitis B vaccine manufactured by recombinant DNA technology, which offers long-term protection against infection, is useful for both preexposure and post-exposure protection, and is the only type currently manufactured in the United States. The other is hepatitis B immune globulin, or HBIG, which is a preparation made from human blood plasma that contains a significant amount of the antibody for the HBV virus. This treatment is indicated, as we will see later, only for temporary protection in certain postexposure situations. It is no longer produced in the United States.

There are two versions of the recombinant hepatitis B vaccine currently in use. The first was licensed in the United States in 1986, and was the first vaccine produced by recombinant DNA technology ever to be approved. In 1989 a second, similar vaccine was cleared for use. The vaccine is made using yeast—the same kind you make bread with—into which the gene for the HBV antibody is inserted. These altered yeast cells then produce HBsAg, the hepatitis B antigen, which is collected and purified. When the process is complete, there is no yeast DNA detectable in the product. You can't get HBV infection from the vaccine, because no infectious viral DNA or complete viral particles are present in the finished vaccine. The vaccine gives an adequate antibody response in 90 percent of healthy adults and 95 percent of kids and adolescents.

The hepatitis B vaccine is administered in three separate doses by a shot in the shoulder for adults or the thigh for infants. For some reason, the vaccine works much better if you get it in your shoulder muscle rather than your rear end, so that is the way it must be given. The second dose is given one month after the first, and the third dose six months after that—this schedule is used for adults and children alike, but the doses vary by age. For hemodialysis patients, or those with compromised immune systems, this schedule has to be adjusted by health care workers and larger doses given. The table below shows the recommended dose of the two vaccines. (As long as they are used at the right doses, it doesn't matter which brand of vaccine you get at any of the three inoculations.)

Recommended doses of currently licensed hepatitis B vaccines

	Dose (in micrograms)	
Group	Recombivax HB*	Engerix-B*
All infants (regardless of whether the mother tests positive for HBV) and children from birth to age 19	5	10
Adults over 20 years old	10	20
Dialysis patients and other immunocompromised people	40†	40§

*Both vaccines are routinely administered in a three-dose series, 0, 1, and 6 months. Engerix-B has also been licensed for a four-dose series administered at 0, 1, 2, and 6 months.

†Special formulation (40 micrograms in 1 ml).

§Two 1 ml doses given at one site, in a four-dose schedule at 0, 1, 2, 6 months.

The complete series includes three shots, but even one dose confers a certain amount of immunity, so even if you think, for example, that it will be tough to get your teenager to show up at the doctor's office for three shots, it's worth starting him or her anyway. And the schedule of doses can vary as well. For adults and children, doses at zero, one, and six months is the usual procedure, but doses at zero, one, and four months or at zero, two, and four months are also effective. Even if the reluctant teenager shows up as much as nine months after the first dose, the second dose can be given at that time and the third two to six months later. There is no circumstance under which the vaccination series should be started over again—even if there is a considerable delay, you can pick up where you left off. Infants, however, should not receive the final dose before they are six months old. In fact, if an infant has been given the third dose before six months, it should be repeated when the infant reaches that age.

Even pregnant or lactating women have taken the vaccine without fear of harming their babies. Of course, you should consult your physician before deciding to take this or any other vaccine. Studies have shown that the vaccination poses no risk to a fetus—but HBV infection in the mother poses considerable risk to the fetus. Pregnant women, including those who have been vaccinated, are now routinely screened for hepatitis B, because a woman could have been infected before she was vaccinated. Only 0.5 percent of all pregnant women test positive for the infection, but all women have to be screened to find that small percentage.

If a person is found to be a carrier of hepatitis B, everyone in their household should be vaccinated. Sexual partners should be tested to see if they are infected, and they should be aware that the vaccine provides a high level of postexposure protection as well.

Although babies now receive HBV vaccine routinely, it can be started at any age. You can get the vaccine from your own doctor, or in a clinic. Your city's public health department can tell you where the vaccine is available, and many city health departments offer the vaccine free of charge. If you have to pay for it, the price varies widely, so shopping around is a good idea. The size of the dose varies by age, and so can the price, so when you're comparing prices you should specify the age of the person receiving the shots.

Side Effects of the Vaccine

The vaccine has very few side effects of any kind—pain at the injection site and elevated temperature are the most common, but both occur just as often with placebo injections. With the less commonly used plasma version of the vaccine, a small number of cases of a neurological disorder called Guillain-Barré syndrome have been reported, but none have been reported with the recombinant version of the vaccine. People with moderate to severe illness should not be vaccinated until their conditions improve, but if you have only a cold or a minor upper respiratory infection you can still be vaccinated safely. Since the vaccine contains no virus, it can be given even to people with compromised immune systems, such as those suffering from HIV infection.

There have been some rare cases of severe adverse reaction to the vaccine. There is, for example, an estimated incidence of 1 in 600,000 doses distributed of anaphylaxis, a severe allergic reaction that impairs breathing and can cause a dramatic drop in blood pressure. There have been isolated case reports of multiple sclerosis, optic neuritis, rheumatoid arthritis, type I diabetes, autoimmune disease, and hair loss following vaccination, but no studies have connected these occurrences to the vaccine. In any case it is clear that the risk of not getting the vaccine—HBV infection, liver disease, and death—is vastly greater than the risk of getting the shots. The CDC estimates that without immunization an extra 2,000 to 5,000 deaths would occur each year from HBV-related liver disease.

A New Baby and Hepatitis B

Darlene Wu was a young Asian woman in the ninth month of her first pregnancy. Her obstetrician had drawn routine bloods, and Ms. Wu's hepatitis B surface antigen and core antibody tests had come back positive. She was visibly upset.

She sat down and I tried to help her relax by chatting about pregnancies and children. But she was there to find out about hepatitis B, and that was the only discussion that could help relieve her anxiety.

"Ms. Wu, I've spoken with Dr. Darnton and she sent me over copies of your blood tests. As she told you, the tests show that you carry the hepatitis B virus. Fortunately, the tests of your liver function are totally normal, and there's no indication that there's been any significant damage to your liver."

She interrupted: "But several of my family members in Taiwan have died of liver disease or liver cancer. And Dr. Darnton said something about transmitting it to my baby. I think I'd die if I gave my baby a disease. And how did I get hepatitis anyway?"

I was sure that we needed to talk about the baby first. Without getting some information and reassurance, she wasn't going to be able to discuss her own situation.

"Let's talk about the baby for a minute. It's true that hepatitis B can be transmitted from a mother to her child. But what's so important in your case is that we know in advance that you have hepatitis B, so we can take steps to protect the baby. It's one of the reasons that your decision to get good prenatal care was just the right thing to do. We can start giving a vaccine to the baby right after birth, and can almost guarantee that he or she won't get hepatitis. You're doing all you can to make sure that your baby is healthy, and you really don't have to worry."

I could see her begin to relax. "As for yourself, there's nothing to worry about for now. Pregnancy can sometimes put a strain on the liver, but there's every indication that you're totally healthy. There are treatments for hepatitis B, and you should definitely consider taking one of them. But that's for sometime in the future, after you've had the baby. In fact, the treatment should wait until after you're done breast-feeding if you plan on it. We'll watch you carefully, and as long as your tests are okay, we'll probably wait until you and the baby have gotten to know each other for a while before we consider your treatment. Does that make sense?"

She indicated that it did, but still wanted to know how she had gotten hepatitis B.

"I don't think I'm going to be able to give you a definite answer," I said, "but let me ask you some questions."

Ms. Wu told me that she had been born in Taiwan. Her parents were still alive, and, as far as she knew, did not have hepatitis. Her mother, however, had been complaining of her abdomen and legs swelling over the past year or so. Ms. Wu had never had blood transfusions, used injection drugs, or had sexual partners other than her husband. Her husband had no history of hepatitis, and she was sure he had never used drugs or had sex with men.

I responded, "As I said, I can't be sure. It may be that your mother does have hepatitis, and that you were infected at birth. That's very common in a number of Asian countries. And people who get hepatitis B at birth often become carriers themselves but don't develop symptoms for many years. That explanation might also account for the swelling that your mother is complaining about—sometimes liver disease can cause swelling of the legs and abdomen. You should suggest that she go to a doctor and have her liver checked out.

"It's also possible that you weren't infected at birth but got hepatitis B later in your childhood. That's also common in countries that have a lot of hepatitis B. Again, just like a baby who's infected, a child will often become a healthy carrier."

Ms. Wu definitely appeared more relaxed and engaged in our discussion. "Let me ask you a question if I may: If I'm a healthy carrier, why should I even bother with being treated?"

"That's a good question. The quick answer is that even healthy carriers of hepatitis B have an increased risk of developing serious liver disease, including cirrhosis and liver cancer. Treatment can sometimes help the body clear out the hepatitis B virus completely, or at least decrease the chance of serious complications.

"I'd like you to get some other blood tests that will help us assess just how active the hepatitis is. They're called hepatitis B e antigen and hepatitis B DNA. And, I'd like your husband to arrange to come in and see me at some point, so we can test him for hepatitis as well."

Vaccinating Infants

Current practice demands that all infants be routinely inoculated with the HBV vaccine. Infants should get three doses, one at birth or within two months of birth, the second one to three months later, and the third two to seventeen months after that. It is likely that the best results are achieved when the final two doses are spaced at least four months apart, but if this schedule is difficult to achieve, then the vaccine can be scheduled along with other childhood vaccines at two-month intervals between doses. The table below shows the various choices for kids born to mothers who are not infected with HBV.

Recommended dosing schedule for hepatitis B vaccine in infants

Hepatitis B vaccine	Age of infant
Option 1	
Dose 1	Before hospital discharge
Dose 2	1–2 months*
Dose 3	6–18 months*
Option 2	
Dose 1	1–2 months*
Dose 2	4 months*
Dose 3	6–18 months*

*Hepatitis B vaccine can be administered simultaneously with diphtheria-tetanus-pertussis, *Haemophilus influenzae* type b conjugate, measles-mumps-rubella, and oral polio vaccines at the same visit.

After You Are Vaccinated

After you get the HBV vaccine, your level of antibodies will decrease with time, but you will still be protected for up to eleven years following immunization. Even after that time, you are still protected against significant—that is, clinically apparent—disease. If you respond to the vaccine—that is, if you produce antibodies—there is very little likelihood that you will ever suffer from HBV. Booster shots are not currently recommended. Studies have followed large numbers of people vaccinated in HBV endemic areas for up to fifteen years, and there has been almost no occurrence of late chronic HBV infections. These studies are continuing. Hemodialysis patients, however, do need booster shots, and the doses of those shots have to be determined by annual testing of the level of antibodies in the blood.

Sometimes the vaccine doesn't work—that is, it doesn't produce the expected antibodies in the blood. This is rare, but when it happens, the person should be vaccinated again. Among "nonresponders," as they are called, an additional dose does the trick for 15 to 20 percent of them, and an additional three doses produce the desired result in 30 to 50 percent. Certain factors are associated with the failure to respond to the HBV vaccine: if you're male, over forty, obese, a smoker, or have a chronic illness, you may not respond as well as other people, but of course the vast majority of people even in these groups respond to the vaccine.

Exposure without Vaccination

What if you are exposed to HBV and haven't had the vaccination? The vaccine works as prophylaxis after exposure, too, provided it is given quickly enough. With infants born to HBV-positive women, the procedure is to give hepatitis B immune globulin (HBIG)—a preparation made from the plasma of pooled donated blood with a high level of HBV antibodies—and the first of the three hepatitis B vaccinations within twelve hours of birth, and then vaccinate the child according to the regular schedule. Other childhood vaccinations can go on normally after the administration of HBIG.

If you are the sexual partner of someone whom you learn has acute hepatitis B and you haven't yourself been vaccinated, you should get the vaccination series and, in addition, a single dose of HBIG. This should be started within fourteen days of the sexual contact.

If you have a percutaneous or mucosal exposure to blood that contains, or even might contain, the virus, you should speak to your doctor about getting the vaccine. If the blood is known to be infected, you should also discuss getting a dose of HBIG within one week after the exposure.

If an unvaccinated infant has a primary caregiver who has acute hepatitis B, the child should get a single dose of HBIG, and then complete the hepatitis B vaccination schedule.

If you are exposed to HBV accidentally as a child or adult, the proper procedure for prophylaxis varies depending on whether you yourself have the protective HBV antibody (HBsAb), and on the HBV status of the source of the contamination (whether that blood is HBsAg positive or not). The following table describes the various situations and recommended procedures.

Chronic Hepatitis B

If you have HBV for six months, you are chronically infected (a carrier), but since you can have HBV without any symptoms, the only way to truly know if you are chronically infected is to have a blood test. The blood

Prophylaxis of HBV infection following accidental exposure through the skin

Exposed person	Treatment when source is:			
	HBsAg positive	HBsAg negative	Not tested or unknown	
Unvaccinated	Give HBIG followed by HBV vaccine	Give HBV vaccine	Give HBV vaccine	
Vaccinated and known to have had an adequate response to the vaccine	Test exposed person for level of antibodies. If it's adequate, no further treatment. If it's not adequate, give HBV vaccine in a booster dose.	No treatment	No treatment	
Vaccinated, but known *not* to have had an adequate response to the vaccine.	Give 2 doses of HBIG or one dose of HBIG and the HBV vaccine	No treatment	If the source is known to be in a high-risk group, treat as if source were HBV infected.	
Response unknown	Test exposed person for level of antibodies. If it's adequate, no further treatment. If it's not adequate, give one dose of HBIG plus the HBV vaccine in a booster dose.	No treatment	Test exposed person for level of antibodies. If it's adequate, no further treatment. If it's not adequate, give HBV vaccine in a booster dose.	

test is easy to get—if you donate blood, for example, the blood bank will test for HBV—but, like everything else about hepatitis, interpreting the test is complicated. It isn't just a question of "you got it or you don't."

There are three standard blood tests for HBV. The first is to see if HBsAg (hepatitis B surface antigen) is present in your blood. If it is, then you are presently HBV infected and you are able to pass the disease on to others.

The second test is for the presence of anti-HBc or HBcAb (antibody to the hepatitis B core antigen). If this is present, it indicates that you have had contact with the HBV virus. But this test is very difficult to interpret, and often results in false positives. What it means often depends on the results of the other two tests.

The third is the test for the anti-HBs or HBsAb (the antibody to hepatitis B surface antigen). If this is positive, it means you have had HBV (or the vaccine for it) and you are immune to the disease. You can't pass it on to other people.

If a blood bank finds positive results on either of the first two tests, that's all they need to know—they won't accept your blood. But you have to know more: you have to know exactly which test you tested positive for. The chart below summarizes the interpretation of the HBV blood test results.

Needless to say (but we'll say it anyway), you can't interpret these results by yourself. A doctor must interpret them for you, and he or she may want to do further blood tests before deciding on a course of action.

When you donate blood, your blood must by law be tested for HBsAg by a specific, quite sensitive FDA-approved method. If the first test is "nonreactive"—that is, if it shows no HBsAg, then your blood will be used (provided all other requirements are met). But if the first

Interpretation of hepatitis B blood test results

Tests	Results	Interpretation
HBsAg	Negative	The person has never been
Anti-HBc	Negative	infected and is susceptible to
Anti-HBs	Negative	hepatitis B.
HBsAg	Negative	Person is immune (safe) and
Anti-HBc	Negative or positive	will not develop HBV
Anti-HBs	Positive	infection again.
		Person is currently infected,
HBsAg	Positive	either acutely or as a hepatitis
Anti-HBc	Positive	B carrier. Test should be
Anti-HBs	Negative	repeated.
HBsAg	Negative	
Anti-HBc	Positive	Multiple interpretations
Anti-HBs	Negative	possible.*

*These are the possible interpretations:

1. The person is recovering from a recent HBV infection. This is rare.

2. The person is distantly immune and the test is not sensitive enough to detect a very low level of anti-HBs.

3. The person is uninfected, and this is a false-positive anti-HBc. This is true about 80 percent of the time.

4. The person has an undetectable level of HbsAg present in the blood and is actually a carrier. This is extremely rare.

test is "reactive" for the antibody, the test will be performed twice more. If both tests are nonreactive, the blood can be used. But if either or both tests are reactive, the unit of blood cannot be used. Before you are notified of the result, one more test will be performed, just to make sure. If this test shows HBsAg, then you will be informed that you cannot donate blood, now or ever. The CDC recommends that this information be presented to you in a sealed letter or in a face-to-face interview. You will be informed in the interview or the letter that you might have chronic HBV, and that you might be infectious to others. You will be told about the vaccine that is available for your household members or sexual partners. Finally, the letter or interviewer will suggest medical follow-up and tell you where you can get it.

If it is determined that you are a carrier, you should see a doctor immediately, and then once every six months after that. The doctor will want to do several things. First, he'll test your blood once again. Sometimes this test will come up negative, indicating that there was a transient acute infection. Then he will want to run the test to determine whether you have the chronic or acute variety of the illness. The doctor will be most interested in seeing how your liver is functioning, since this is the organ that the HBV virus attacks and destroys. You can see your regular doctor, but you will also want to consult with a gastroenterologist, preferably an expert in hepatology, the subspecialty that deals with diseases of the liver. You will want to avoid alcohol, which can cause liver damage. And you will have to inform your doctor of any medicines you are taking, including over-the-counter drugs, because many drugs can cause stress to the liver. As long as you remain a "healthy carrier," which could be the rest of your life, this will be your procedure.

Recovery from Hepatitis B

Robert looked a bit like Woody Allen, but with a spiky crewcut. He gave me a warm smile as I asked him to take a seat and tell me how he was feeling.

"I feel fine, but I figure it's time for me to get a complete exam. I'm forty-five, and I finally got a job that has decent health insurance. And I'd like part of the exam to be an HIV test."

I assured him that that was fine and asked him why he thought HIV was a possibility.

He laughed. "I'm a very gay guy, and although I've been using condoms regularly for years, I wasn't always so safe. I have no symptoms, but I've never been tested."

Since we were already discussing sexually transmitted diseases, I finished that part of the history and found out that Robert had had rectal gonorrhea twice when he was in his twenties. He had also had mononucleosis at about the same time. The rest of his history and his physical were unremarkable. I ordered routine studies and an HIV test.

He came back two weeks later for the results. His HIV test was negative, but his liver serologies were not. His hepA IgG antibodies were positive, indicating that he had had hepatitis A sometime in the past. No problem. His hepC antibody study was negative. Fine. His hepatitis B tests were not as good: his hepatitis B surface antigen and core antibody were positive, indicating that he was a hepatitis B carrier. His ALT was almost three times the upper limits of normal.

We went over the results, and I asked him to think back to any time that he might have had acute hepatitis. When he repeated that the only time in his life that he had felt sick for any period of time was when he had mononucleosis, I asked him to describe his symptoms at that time. He said he had felt awful—achy, tired, and nauseated for several weeks. He had had some diarrhea. He didn't remember his eyes being yellow or his stool light-colored. He also denied having had a sore throat, a striking symptom in most cases of mono. He didn't remember the college doctor taking any blood tests; the doctor just told him that he had mononucleosis and to take it easy. The symptoms could easily have been due to either hepatitis A or B. When I asked him if he had been sexually active at that time, Robert got a gleam in his eye and told me that college was the time when he had discovered his own sexuality and also discovered Greenwich Village. He had been very active during that period.

I explained that I needed to get some confirmatory tests, but that he should assume he was truly positive. I assured him that there were treatments available, and that we would discuss them further when the tests came back. In the meanwhile, I explained, I strongly advised him to stay away from alcohol. He wanted to know if marijuana was a problem, and I told him that there was no evidence that it injured the liver, but that he was smart enough to know the other potential problems (legal and otherwise) it could cause. I asked him if he would advise his current and former lovers to have themselves checked for hepatitis and to get the hepatitis B vaccine if they were negative. He knew about the precautions to be taken to avoid transmission of HIV through blood, semen, or other body fluids, and I told him to apply all those lessons to hepatitis B.

His hepatitis B DNA and e antigen were both positive, signifying active and rapid viral replication. I told him that I thought he was a good candidate for interferon treatment, but that the decision was truly his. Many people who are carriers live out a normal life without developing serious liver disease or liver cancer, and he might certainly be one of those. On the other hand, the fact that his enzymes were elevated and the viral DNA and e antigen were positive put him at some real risk of these serious complications.

He interrupted to say that he definitely wanted to be treated. I explained that the interferon was effective less often than not, and that it had some serious side effects. And assuming it did not work in sixteen weeks, he would need to take lamivudine for at least a year thereafter. My description of the possible side effects from interferon slowed him down a bit, but he still decided he wanted to proceed.

Robert was great about giving himself the injections three times a week. He missed two weeks of work during the first month of treatment because of flulike symptoms. He was upset when some of his hair began to fall out, but he persevered. After sixteen weeks his ALT was normal but a repeat e antigen was still positive. He started on lamivudine and had no side effects.

A year later, Robert was one of those lucky patients who revert to being e antigen negative with a nondetectable DNA. He stopped the lamivudine and comes to see me every six months. His prognosis is excellent.

Living with Chronic HBV

About 10 percent of adults infected with HBV become carriers. Children have a greater risk, and the earlier they are infected, the greater the chance that they will be lifelong carriers of the virus. Sometimes, though rarely, HBV carriers will clear the infection from their bodies, but most will not. Usually carriers lead healthy normal lives, but they are at considerably greater risk for liver failure and liver cancer. Chronic HBV has a variable course—some people suffer very little liver damage; others progress to cirrhosis and hepatocellular carcinoma (liver cancer).

If you do develop liver disease, you have to take extra precautions. You should get a flu vaccination every year, and, if you have severe illness, a pneumococcal vaccine as well. Hepatitis A can also harm your liver, so you have to be vaccinated against that disease. And you must not eat raw oysters, because they may carry *Vibrio vulnificus,* which can cause septicemia in people with liver disease. This septicemia is fatal 40 percent of the time.

If you are a carrier, even if you feel healthy, you can infect others, so you have to take precautions to make sure this doesn't happen. Blood, semen, and vaginal fluids carry the virus, and contact with these bodily fluids can transmit the virus to others. Although the virus can be found in saliva in low concentrations, there is no evidence that it can be transmitted by contact with saliva unless a bite has occurred. Kissing, or contact with a drooling infant, for example, has never been shown to be a mode of transmission. Sweat, tears, urine, and respiratory secretions do not carry the virus.

Rules for HBV Carriers

- Cover any cuts or open sores with a bandage.
- Discard used personal items such as tampons, tissues, or bandages in a paper bag.
- Wash your hands after touching any bodily fluids.
- Clean up blood spills with bleach—one part household bleach to ten parts water.
- Tell your sexual partners that you are infected so that they can be tested. If your sexual partner(s) is not immune, he or she should have the vaccination series and be tested one to two months after the last dose to make sure he or she is protected.
- Use condoms.
- Have your household members tested for HBV.
- Tell your doctors that you are a carrier.

- If you are pregnant, your doctor must know your HBV status, because your baby must be started on hepatitis B prophylaxis shortly after birth.
- Don't share chewing gum, razors, toothbrushes, or washcloths with anyone else.
- Don't share needles used for tattooing or body piercing, or any other equipment that touches your blood or infectious body fluids.
- Don't chew food for your baby.
- Don't donate blood, plasma, body organs, tissue, or sperm.

The Treatment of Chronic HBV

In assessing a case of HBV infection, doctors divide the disease into four stages, defined by the presence or absence of various disease markers—the antigens, antibodies, DNA markers, and enzyme levels that characterize the illness. These include HBsAg, the antibody to HBsAg, HBV DNA, the antibody to HBcAg, HBeAg, and the antibody to HBeAg. ALT and AST tests are also considered in deciding what stage the disease is in. Determining the stage of the disease is essential to deciding on treatment. Of the four stages of illness, summarized in the chart below, treatment is only effective in stage 2, and the goal is to move from stage 2 to stage 3; that is, to stop replication of the virus, a state indicated by the absence of the antigen HBeAg and the presence of the antibody to it.

Interferon

If you have chronic HBV it's too late for the vaccine, but you can still be treated for the illness. Current practice dictates that patients who are hepatitis B surface anti-

Stages of HBV infection

Disease marker	Stage 1	Stage 2	Stage 3	Stage 4
HBsAg	Positive	Positive	Positive	Negative
Antibody to HBsAg	Negative	Negative	Negative	Positive
HBV DNA	Negative	Negative	Negative	Positive
Antibody to HBcAg	Positive	Positive	Positive	Positive
HbeAg	Positive	Positive	Negative	Negative
Antibody to HBeAg	Negative	Negative	Positive	Positive
Aspartate and alanine aminotransferase (AST and ALT) levels	Normal	Elevated	Normal	Normal

gen positive, HBV DNA negative, and have elevated ALT blood levels—that is, those in stage 2 of the illness—are candidates for treatment with interferon. Most of these patients will also be hepatitis B e antigen (HBeAg) positive, but some may not be. Treatment in other stages doesn't do much good, and treatment of people with advanced liver disease can be dangerous and actually speed the process of liver deterioration. Rates of progression of the disease are highly variable from one person to another, depending on the state of the immune system, the age of the person, the stage of the infection, and geographical and genetic factors.

Interferon is expensive, its use is difficult, and treatment with it is fraught with problematic side effects. This makes deciding who will most benefit from it very important. Although many people with hepatitis B (and their doctors) will want to try anything that holds any promise for a cure, there are some patients who clearly respond better to interferon treatment than others. People with low levels of HBV DNA, high AST levels, a shorter duration of hepatitis infection, and heterosexual orientation appear to respond best. Those who were infected as children and those in groups where transmission from mothers to children is common respond poorly. The level of HBV DNA is the most sensitive predictor: in a large clinical trial, patients with levels of less than 100 mg/ml had a 50 percent response rate; those with levels of greater than 200 mg/ml had a response rate of 7 percent, no different from that of the untreated control group.

The reasons for these varying responses to therapy have to do with the condition of the immune system. Low HBV DNA and high AST levels indicate that the immune system is fighting the infection actively. Children exposed at birth develop a tolerant response, treating the virus as if it were an ordinary part of their biological makeup, rather than a foreign invader. Their immune systems don't put up a fight against the virus, and they respond poorly to interferon treatment.

First, you should have tests to assess your liver status (liver function tests, and other blood tests, are described in the appendix). But the real goal is to stop the virus from reproducing, and there are tests to determine if this is happening as treatment progresses. Any evidence of liver cancer should be looked for, and, although there is some debate about how best to monitor this problem, it is reasonable to have an ultrasound and alpha-fetoprotein estimation (alpha-fetoprotein is a chemical marker for cancerous tumors) every six months. If you are not immune to hepatitis A, you should be vaccinated for it. Your family members and sexual partners should be tested and vaccinated against hepatitis B as soon as possible, even if pregnant. If there is evidence from the blood tests that you are suffering liver disease, a liver biopsy will probably be necessary to get a complete picture of the health of your liver. We say "probably" necessary because the value of this expensive and rather uncomfortable procedure has not been fully analyzed for cost-effectiveness.

Interferon is a protein manufactured by various cells in your body, including the cells of the liver, to fight off disease. In 1992 the FDA approved a synthesized, genetically engineered version of this substance for use in the treatment of viral infections. Unfortunately, only about 15 to 20 percent of chronic HBV patients will have a lasting response to interferon.

Interferon is not easy to use. It must be injected either into a muscle or under the skin, and the shots must be given daily or at least three times a week for several months. To use the drug, you have to learn to give yourself injections. Also, it has unpleasant side effects—fever, muscle aches, chills, fatigue, and diarrhea are among the minor ones. Some are more serious: suicidal thoughts, numbness in the extremities, irregular heartbeat, trouble concentrating. If you have any of these more serious symptoms, you should tell your doctor about them immediately. These side effects tend to diminish as therapy progresses, however, so you shouldn't let them discourage you from taking a promising treatment.

Within four to six months of treatment, 30 to 40 percent of patients clear HBV from their blood as measured by non-PCR assays. Often the rates of clearance continue to increase after treatment is stopped. Because of side effects, about one-quarter of patients have to have their doses reduced during treatment.

So does interferon work or not? Studies have shown

that the drug does eliminate detectable HBsAg (hepatitis B surface antigen) in some patients, but only a minority. About half of patients will have a reduction in HBeAg or in hepatitis B virus DNA. And when HBeAg is cleared after treatment with interferon, these patients have a better clinical outcome. But it would be wrong to say that this constitutes a cure. The fact remains that interferon therapy is successful only in patients who have the proper immune response. And since you can't predict with certainty which patients these will be, you have to treat a large number of people in order to cure some of them.

Lamivudine

The newest treatment for chronic HBV is the antiviral drug lamivudine, sometimes called 3TC, which is also used for treating HIV. It is given in 100 mg pills once a day, and can be used for up to a year with minimal side effects. No one knows whether taking lamivudine for more than a year is safe or effective.

Studies have shown that after one to three months of treatment with this drug, HBV DNA is cleared from the blood of almost all patients, but only about one-fifth of them have sustained results. The same appears to be true with treatment as long as one year. Most initially get better, in the sense that their HBV DNA is undetectable, but the majority have a recurrence when treatment is stopped. Part of the problem may be that mutant strains of the virus begin to appear after about six months of treatment, even though the mutant strains are usually less virulent than the original HBV virus. Little is known about how to treat such infections, or whether larger doses of lamivudine would prevent them. In clinical trials, patients who developed mutant strains were less responsive to treatment than those who did not.

Lamivudine is not believed to work through an immune mechanism—that is, unlike interferon, it does not stimulate the body's own immune system. Nevertheless, those with an active immune system response to the virus (that is, those with low HBV DNA and high AST levels) seem to respond better to lamivudine.

Famciclovir

This drug has been used successfully to treat herpes simplex virus infection and varicella zoster virus (shingles), and it also seems to suppress HBV replication in some patients. Since famciclovir attacks a different region of the HBV virus, it may be possible to use lamivudine and famciclovir together as a more effective medicine and one less likely to produce drug-resistant viral strains. But famciclovir, unlike lamivudine, is not currently approved as a treatment for HBV. The results of ongoing clinical trials will have to be assessed first. For now, treatment with interferon is the first line of attack, and lamivudine is reserved for patients who fail to respond to interferon. Like many other facets of clinical practice in treating viral diseases, this approach will undoubtedly be modified in the near future.

To Vaccinate or Not to Vaccinate

Many people figure, quite correctly, that they are at very low risk for getting HBV. They don't travel to exotic parts of the world, they only have one sex partner, they don't do drugs, they aren't dialysis patients, they don't get transfusions regularly, they aren't health care workers or otherwise routinely exposed to blood or blood products. In fact, they're right: they probably won't get HBV.

On the other hand, remember that about one-third of

cases of HBV are among people who don't fit into any
of these categories. They don't know how they got it.
The HBV virus is very durable—it lasts for weeks on
environmental surfaces, where, presumably, anyone can
come in contact with it. So although it isn't likely, you
can still get HBV even if you aren't in one of the risk
groups. And as you can see if you've read the description
of chronic HBV above, the illness can be very unpleasant
and difficult to treat.

The vaccine for HBV is totally safe and almost 100
percent effective. It can often be had for free. It involves
three relatively painless shots in the arm. It has almost no
side effects, and what side effects it has are minor. So the
question becomes: Would you rather have the three shots
and no risk of the disease, or skip the shots and have a
small risk? There will be differing answers to this question, but most doctors would answer this way: Take the
shots and avoid the risk completely.

There is a further reason to get the vaccine. HBV
vaccine has been available since 1982, but it has had almost no effect in eradicating the illness. This is because
the initial vaccination programs targeted high-risk groups
only, and that turned out not to be enough to get rid of
this very durable virus. So it was that in 1991 the American Council on Immunization Practices recommended
universal vaccination of newborns and adolescents. The
HBV vaccination program has not so far been met with
great enthusiasm by physicians, but cooperation with it
may help eliminate an expensive, debilitating, and sometimes deadly disease.

4

Hepatitis C

THE BASIC FACTS ABOUT
THE VIRUS

Doctors knew the symptoms of hepatitis long before they knew exactly what caused them. By the 1930s scientists knew that there were two kinds of hepatitis—infectious hepatitis, transmitted largely by food or water, and serum hepatitis, transmitted by contact with blood. While they could distinguish these two diseases clinically, no one knew what organism was involved. Although the beliefs about the means of transmission of the two diseases would later have to be revised somewhat (as you know if you have read the previous two chapters of this book), it was eventually discovered that there were two different viruses causing these illnesses, later designated hepatitis A (infectious hepatitis) and hepatitis B (serum hepatitis). The virus that causes hepatitis B was isolated in the 1960s, and by 1973 the virus that causes hepatitis A was also discovered.

A New Kind of Hepatitis

Then, starting in the 1970s, doctors began to notice a disease they hadn't seen before. It looked like hepatitis, with symptoms very much like those of hepatitis A and hepatitis B, and the same kind of liver involvement. While it seemed to have a more chronic course than either HAV or HBV, it was still clearly some kind of hepatitis. But when patients with this disease had their blood tested, neither hepatitis A nor hepatitis B showed up. So physicians began calling the new disease "non-A, non-B hepatitis." It was noticed fairly early on that this disease was transmitted in blood transfusions. In fact, about 10 percent of people who got frequent transfusions— hemophiliacs, for example—would come down with some kind of liver inflammation, often the non-A, non-B disease, but there was nothing anyone could find in the blood supply that would account for the problem. The increases were also noticed in Japan, where rising rates of cirrhosis made people suspect that some pathogen might be the cause.

There were other hints. Studies showed that injection drug users, health care workers, people who lived with hepatitis sufferers, and people with many sexual partners were all at higher risk for developing this new kind of hepatitis. There was no question that there was something being carried in blood that was moving from one person to another.

In the late 1980s scientists began closing in on the virus. Using serum from a person infected with non-A, non-B hepatitis, they were able to cause the mysterious disease in a chimpanzee (chimps and tamarin monkeys are the only other species known to be susceptible to the disease). So they knew they had infected blood. Next they extracted blood from the animal and isolated the plasma. Then they centrifuged the infectious plasma, spinning out a tiny pellet that contained the viral particles and nucleic acids.

The next step was to "denature" the proteins—break them into their component parts. Organisms called phages can pick up these small bits of nucleic acid and express them on their surfaces. This creates a "library" of all the different genetic materials found in the original sample. These phages were then cloned to make many copies of the "books" in the phage library.

Then the researchers took blood from two chimps, one that had been exposed to non-A, non-B hepatitis and one that had not been, and tagged all the antibodies from the two samples with chemical markers so that they could be identified.

Finally, they put the tagged antibodies from the uninfected sample into plates holding one copy of the entire phage library, and antibodies from the infected sample into another copy of the library. They then compared the two, and found that antibodies from the infected sample attached to one more phage clone than the antibodies from the uninfected sample. This showed that there was an expression of viral proteins from the infected sample that did not appear in the uninfected sample. Later they found that the protein was an RNA virus. By identifying the unique antibody, the researchers could develop a screening test for the HCV infection.

For the first time, a molecular biological technique—the cloning of nucleic acid—had been used to identify a disease agent that had never been seen, cultured, or defined by the antibodies that attack it. Because these researchers worked for a profit-making company, one of the first things they did when they found the virus was to patent it.

The stock of the company, Chiron, shot up immediately because people hoped that a profitable vaccine would soon follow. But now, more than ten years later, little more than diagnostic blood tests for the virus have been produced, and, like many stocks that soar on promises of unrealized "scientific breakthroughs," Chiron's has settled back to former levels. But research goes on at Chiron and in other places. One of the large problems faced by those trying to develop a drug treatment for HCV is that the virus thrives and reproduces inside the cell rather than on its surface, and it is very difficult to design a drug that will penetrate the cell wall. But it's not impossible—the protease inhibitors that have revolutionized the treatment of HIV are an example of a "small molecule" drug that does this.

The Structure and Life Cycle of the Hepatitis C Virus

Hepatitis C is a flavivirus, a member of the same family as the viruses that cause yellow fever and dengue fever. Like those viruses, it has a genome that consists of a single strand of RNA.

When a hepatitis C virus enters your bloodstream, it seeks out a liver cell. This is the only place in your body where it can reproduce. One particular protein on its shell, called the E2 protein, attaches itself to the outside of a liver cell at a place called a receptor site. Then the protein core of the virus penetrates the cell's wall. It does this chemically, by merging its lipid coat with the cell wall. Once fused like this, the cell wall surrounds and engulfs the virus, bringing it inside. Now inside the cell, the virus can release its load of viral RNA and begin its work of reproducing its genetic material.

Inside the cell, the virus's coat dissolves and releases viral RNA that then takes over parts of the cell—the ribosomes—to manufacture the material it needs for reproduction. In a sense, the virus "fools" the cell into treating the viral RNA as if it were its own. During this process, the virus either shuts down the normal functions of the cell or forces it to make more infected cells (which may be why the virus is associated with liver cancer). Now the viral RNA begins to copy itself billions of times, creating the material for new viruses. The large number of reproductive processes going on gives ample opportunity for genetic mutations, creating the RNA for new strains and subtypes of the hepatitis C virus. An infected person can produce 1,000 billion copies of hepatitis C virus per day.

Finally, the viral RNA creates capsomeres, the stuff of which the virus's protein coat is made. These capsomeres fit together like building blocks, eventually forming a shell called a capsid. This material encapsulates the viral RNA in a spherical form, creating a new virus. The liver cell cooperates by providing the virus with a protective lipid coat and then releasing it to start the cycle all over again, attacking another liver cell. This goes on repeatedly at the cell's surface, until the cell dies.

The process includes the production of certain enzymes, called protease, helicase, and polymerase enzymes, that are essential in the virus's reproduction. The structure of these enzymes is well-known, and this knowledge is the first step in designing a drug to attack them and thus interfere with the virus's reproduction.

Worldwide Epidemic

Once a more or less reliable test for HCV was developed, the extent of the problem could be examined, and the results were startling: hepatitis C was everywhere, no matter what population was screened. Estimates of worldwide infection are as high as 240 million.

Developing countries have the highest rates, but rates in North America and western Europe are higher than in eastern Europe. Epidemiologists have theorized that the higher rates in the United States might be accounted for by the large number of immigrants from areas of high prevalence, and by the widespread use of illegal injection drugs. American military involvement in Asia during World War II, the Korean War, and the Vietnam War may also be a factor. There is some evidence that cases of liver disease are increasing among patients admitted to Veterans Administration hospitals. The internationalization of the blood supply undoubtedly helped spread the illness as well. The CDC estimates that 300,000 U.S. citizens were exposed via infected blood products before 1992, when screening of blood for HCV antibodies began.

A Trojan Horse

HCV, like HIV, has to be inside the cell before it can replicate. (However, unlike HIV, HCV is not a retrovirus. That is, it does not incorporate its genetic structure into the cell it invades.) In a sense, HCV fools the body's immune system into allowing it to pass through the cell wall, and then once inside starts reproducing and causing disease. And it has another nasty trick: it varies its appearance so that the immune system is constantly faced with new challenges. The virus, in other words, is not a single entity, but a family of viruses with different genetic structures and different subtypes. Various strains of the virus can exist not only in different infected people but even within the same person. This gives the immune system a serious challenge: it must respond not to one virus, but to different forms of the same virus. This multi-pronged attack usually results in victory for the virus, and defeat for the immune system. Scientists now believe that this trick of varying its appearance is what gives the HCV virus the ability to cause such persistent chronic infection, essentially changing its form every time the immune system devises a response to it. Moreover, it may be that, as with HIV, even more new and resistant strains begin to develop when drugs are used to attack HCV.

There are now six large groups of HCV, called types or genotypes, labeled 1 through 6. Each of these genotypes contains many subtypes (more than ninety have been discovered), called 1a, 1b, 2a, 2b, and so on. In North America, most cases—about 70 percent—are 1a or 1b subtypes. The rest are 2, 3, and 4. Type 2 is common in Japan and in China. Type 3 predominates in Europe and the United Kingdom. Type 4 is common in the Middle East and central Africa. Type 5 is rare in North America, but dominates in South Africa. Type 6 is often found in Hong Kong and Macao. Types 1a and 1b seem to cause the most severe disease, and the cases most resistant to treatment. In addition to these genotypes, there are many small variants of the genomes within the genotypes, forms that may multiply over time within the same individual and may also contribute to resistance to drugs.

This kind of genotyping is a research tool, and, at least for the moment, has very little clinical significance.

Type 1 is more resistant to treatment, but in fact you probably can't even find out what genotype of virus you have unless you are in an experimental protocol at a research institution. The genotype or subtype of your HCV infection will probably make little difference in your treatment regimen.

While the virus was isolated in 1989, not until quite recently was it shown that it alone can cause the disease. This required making a tissue culture of the virus, making sure that the organism was purified, and that it was this organism that was causing HCV disease. This is an essential step in finding a treatment.

By 1992, effective methods for detecting HCV in the blood had been developed, and now blood is routinely screened for HCV. Although the risk of getting HCV from a blood transfusion is not zero, it's pretty close: since 1994 the risk for transfusion-transmitted HCV infection has been so low that the CDC has been unable to detect a single case. But people who received transfusions before 1992 are at risk for HCV. And, as we will see later, they may have it without even knowing.

Today, 60 percent of the transmission of HCV can be traced to injection drug use, and, for reasons that are not entirely clear, the dramatic decrease in new cases of HCV began with decreases in new cases among this population. The decline accelerated considerably when blood screening for HCV began in 1992.

Attacking the Liver, and More

Like other forms of hepatitis, HCV enters the bloodstream and moves through the blood to the liver. Here it seeks out liver cells, penetrates their walls, and begins reproducing inside the cells. As your body starts to defend against this attack, the liver becomes inflamed, cells are destroyed, and the functioning of the liver deteriorates. This deterioration doesn't necessarily happen quickly, and in some infections it doesn't happen at all. Many people with chronic HCV infection have no more damage to their livers than anyone else—often people are unaware for years, even decades, that they are carriers of HCV. But others, particularly the elderly, those who have alcoholism or other kinds of hepatitis, and those with HIV, suffer severe liver disease when they are infected with HCV.

Although the virus exerts its most obvious effect on the liver, researchers have recently discovered that it attacks at least one other kind of cell as well: a type of white blood cell called a peripheral blood mononuclear cell. This discovery has convinced many doctors that the disease is a systemic illness, not just a liver ailment, and that this may be one of the reasons it is so difficult to treat.

HCV also almost always infects the lymphatic system as well as the liver. The lymphatic system is part of the body's immune system. It has vessels that run throughout the body, and lymph nodes in the neck, armpits, and groin. Usually, the kind of infection that HCV causes in the lymphatic system is subclinical—that is, it doesn't have any symptoms and doesn't do any harm. But there is a poorly understood association between non-Hodgkin's lymphoma (a cancer of the lymph nodes) and HCV infection. It isn't clear that HCV can actually cause non-Hodgkin's lymphoma, but there is a suspiciously high prevalence of HCV among patients with non-Hodgkin's lymphoma, and lymphatic disease should always be considered as a possible complication of HCV infection.

To complicate matters even further, it is now known

that the HCV virus attacks the body not by directly destroying cells themselves, but by provoking immune responses that cause other kinds of damage. The immune system has two different kinds of attack against viruses. In one, it produces antibodies that destroy the virus by attaching themselves to the proteins on the outside of the virus. These antibodies are very effective in defeating hepatitis A and hepatitis B—so effective that their very presence indicates immunity. But the antibodies produced by the immune system for hepatitis C don't work at all, probably because the hepatitis C virus has so many different kinds of genomes on its surface that the antibodies can't figure out a way to attack it. So instead, the immune system takes another tack: it destroys the liver cells that the virus attacks, using organisms called cytotoxic T lymphocytes. This works well enough, at least for a while, because the liver is good at regenerating itself. But eventually—sometimes after many years—cells near the infected ones start to become inflamed and begin to secrete collagen and other proteins, which gradually cause fibrosis, and finally cirrhosis of the liver.

The virus, in other words, "tells" the body to destroy other cells or initiate harmful biochemical processes of various kinds. The hardening of the liver caused by the disease is generated by this immune response, not by the destruction of the cells themselves. In fact, the presence of the virus may be less significant in causing disease than the immune system response that it provokes. Some people can have very high concentrations of the virus in their bloodstreams without suffering any symptoms, and doctors now believe that the reason this is possible is that the virus, for unknown reasons, fails to provoke the destructive immune system response in these people. That the immune system's reaction is part of the problem in HCV infection has implications for treatment—trying to prevent the immune reaction may be a more successful approach than attacking and killing the virus itself.

About 15 percent of people infected with HCV fight off the virus, recover, and never have it detectable in the blood again. But the rest fail to clear the virus within six months, and are thus classified as chronic carriers of the disease. The course of their illness can vary considerably from one person to another.

Disease with and without Symptoms

The HCV virus is sometimes called "indolent"—that is, you can be infected with it for many years without having any symptoms. The reasons for this are unclear. Some researchers believe that although the virus proliferates rapidly, it can be detected by tests before there are large enough concentrations of it in the blood to produce disease. Others are convinced that the virus reproduces as quickly as any other virus, but makes defective copies of itself that don't do much harm to the patient or don't survive. Or it may be that the body successfully fights off the virus for a time, or somehow manages to destroy some of the virus particles while others "hide" from the immune system.

Viruses are in general very small, but even by these standards the HCV virus is minuscule. Even the best electron micrograph technology can hardly see it, and the one picture of it produced by a team of researchers in Tokyo is not accepted as genuine by everyone. Moreover, even small amounts of this small virus can cause illness. If you imagine that testing for the presence of small amounts of a very small virus would be difficult, you are right. It's expensive too.

The genetic material of HCV virus is RNA—ribonucleic acid. Many viruses have DNA—deoxyribonucleic acid—as their genetic material. When DNA-based viruses reproduce, they usually produce identical copies of themselves. But RNA is less stable, more likely to produce mutations, and so HCV, when it reproduces, can change its genetic makeup quite easily. Thus finding a drug that will track it down and kill it becomes that much more difficult—it keeps finding new disguises to hide behind. And this variability is why there are so many different types and strains of HCV, and why one person can have several different genetic variants of the virus in his bloodstream at the same time.

Signs of HCV Infection

HCV can have many different symptoms at different times during the course of the infection, or it can have no symptoms at all. It is important to remember that the number and severity of symptoms suffered bears little relationship to the amount of liver damage the disease is causing. Below is a list of symptoms that HCV-infected people may suffer. Almost no one suffers all of them, and of course these symptoms can be symptoms of many other diseases besides HCV. No one should conclude that because he has felt some of these symptoms at one time or another, he is therefore infected with HCV. The diagnosis of HCV requires at least a blood test, and usually other diagnostic tools, and the tests require careful interpretation.

- Flulike symptoms—malaise, chills, fever, indigestion, loss of appetite, diarrhea
- Pain in the upper right side of the abdomen beneath the rib cage where the liver is located

- Stomach bloating
- Pain in the joints
- Mood disturbances, mental fatigue or dysfunction, or frequent or continuous headaches
- Chronic or acute periods of exhaustion, and poor sleep patterns
- Bad reactions to alcohol or fatty food
- Fluid retention or puffy face
- Itchy skin
- Swelling of the lymph nodes in the neck, armpits, or groin
- Frequent urination
- Blood sugar disorders
- In women, irregular menses, problems related to menopause, and lower libido
- Chest pains
- Dizziness or vision problems
- Numbness in the extremities

Although these symptoms may occur at some point, very few people notice anything wrong when they first get HCV—even the usual symptoms of hepatitis (jaundice, nausea, and so on) occur in fewer than 5 percent of people who contract HCV. It is extremely rare that anyone dies of an acute HCV infection, although there have been reports of such cases. For the most part, HCV is a chronic condition whose subtle and slowly developing signs make diagnosis difficult and misdiagnosis common. But almost everyone who contracts the infection does eventually develop symptoms of some kind.

Roughly one-fifth of patients will suffer cirrhosis within the first twenty years after infection. For some the damage will stop at this point; for others the damage to the liver gradually gets worse. At the end, when liver disease takes its toll, the patient will suffer from jaundice, accumulation of fluid within the abdomen, bleeding in the esophagus, and mental confusion. Liver cancer is also a risk for hepatitis C infected patients.

A recent study published in the *New England Journal of Medicine* suggests that children who are infected with HCV are more likely to recover than adults. The study examined 458 children who had undergone heart surgery in Germany before blood was routinely screened for HCV. Fifteen percent were infected. After twenty years, however, the disease had cleared completely in half of these people, and among the other half very few had any liver disease. This contrasts with the 20 percent or so of adults who manage to clear the infection completely. No one knows why infected children recover at higher rates than infected adults, and no one knows whether these kids will suffer higher rates of liver disease as time goes on.

Most adults infected with HCV—about 70 percent— experience some liver dysfunction. This can be a very gradual progression of disease, so gradual that the patient grows old and dies of something else before the liver seriously deteriorates; or it can progress within a few years to cirrhosis, liver cancer, and death. What accounts for the very variable progression of the disease may be genetic, may have something to do with lifestyle or environment, or may have multiple causes. No one knows for sure.

Who Has It, and How Did They Get It?

HCV is the most common chronic bloodborne infection in the United States. It isn't completely clear how infectious the disease is—that is, what concentrations of virus in the blood are required for the disease to be transmitted and exactly what kinds of behavior will help transmit it. During the 1980s an average of 230,000 new infections occurred every year, but the rate of new infections began to decline radically in the 1990s. In 1996 there were only 36,000 new infections. Almost four million Americans have been infected with the virus. Of these, most are chronically infected, and many are not even aware that they are infected since they aren't suffering any symptoms. The cost to society in medical expenses and work lost is estimated to be more than $600 million a year, and HCV-associated liver disease is now the most frequent indication for liver transplantation among adults. The future looks bad: because most HCV-infected people are between thirty and fifty years of age, the number of deaths attributable to the disease could increase significantly over the next ten to twenty years as this group reaches the age range when liver disease typically occurs.

An Unlikely Case of Hepatitis C

Stephen Leibniz came in for an initial visit. He appeared to be in his mid-seventies, tall, probably six foot four, and painfully thin. He had a firm handshake and a resounding bass voice.

His problem, he said, was that his legs had begun to swell. In my mind, a differential diagnosis began to form: venous insufficiency (varicose veins) was simplest and most likely, but a man of his age could certainly have heart failure; kidney or liver disease were possible but much less common.

His medical history was straightforward: severe varicose veins that required surgery in his early forties; recurrent duodenal ulcers for which he had part of his stomach removed (an operation no longer performed); and prostate surgery for benign enlargement of the gland in his sixties. He was a longtime heavy smoker, but claimed to have little problem with shortness of breath. He had no clinical history of heart disease.

His physical exam was most notable for what he didn't have: no superficial varicose veins, no abnormal heart sounds, no suggestion of fluid in his lungs. He did have quite a bit of fluid in his legs. I felt for the lymph nodes in the groin, wondering if he could have metastatic prostate cancer that was enlarging and scarring the nodes and causing the lymph fluid to pool in his legs. The lymph nodes and his prostate gland felt normal. The only real surprise was that I was pretty sure I could feel his spleen, and that suggested cirrhosis as a possible diagnosis.

Before he went for the blood tests I ordered, I asked him if he had ever had hepatitis or been a heavy drinker. He gave a simple no to both questions.

The blood tests left little doubt that his liver was the cause of his problem: his AST and ALT were only minimally elevated, but his protein was extremely low. His liver was not producing enough albumin, and as a result fluid was leaking from his bloodstream into the tissues of his legs. The liver serology tests were negative for hepatitis A and B, but positive for hepatitis C. How did this seventy-six-year-old man get a form of hepatitis most associated with injection drug users?

When he came for his follow-up visit, I did a more thorough history. No, he had never injected drugs, but he had had blood transfusions in the mid-1980s. The doctor who did the prostate scraping had hit a blood vessel, causing profuse bleeding that required two units of blood. While I couldn't be sure the transfusions were the cause of the hepatitis C, it certainly made sense.

I explained what I had found and told Mr. Leibniz that I thought he might have cirrhosis. His first reaction was to reassert that he had never been a heavy drinker, but I explained that hepatitis C alone could cause cirrhosis, and could do it without ever making him sick. I did strongly suggest that he avoid any alcohol from now on to protect his liver from additional damage.

I explained that I wanted to verify the diagnosis and do some other tests to assess the stage of his disease. Rechecking for hepC would just require another blood test called a RIBA, but I wanted him to do two other tests: an ultrasound examination of his abdomen and a liver biopsy. The ultrasound was easy—it was like having a microphone rubbed over the abdomen and would show the size of his liver and spleen. The liver biopsy was more complicated since it involved putting a good-sized needlelike device into his liver. A G-I specialist would do the biopsy in a procedures room in the hospital, but if everything went okay, Mr. Leibniz could count on being out the same day.

The ultrasound showed that the liver was relatively small and irregular, the classic finding in cirrhosis. The spleen was enlarged and there was some free fluid (ascites) in the abdominal cavity, both as a result of high pressures in the portal system caused by the scarring in the liver. The liver biopsy confirmed the diagnosis of established cirrhosis.

The discussion with Mr. Leibniz was not easy. Given the extent of the damage to his liver, there was little point in treating him with interferon. I tried to be optimistic in presenting the natural history of cirrhosis: many people live with it for years with only minor problems, like his leg swelling. We would treat that with a diuretic. But I also had to warn him that his blood clotting factors were low due to the liver disease, and he would be more prone to bleeding. I knew that he would have to be watched carefully to see if his liver lost the ability to metabolize proteins effectively; if it did, his blood ammonia level would rise and potentially harm his brain. His portal hypertension could also cause veins in his esophagus to swell (varices), and they could rupture and cause massive bleeding.

In fact, that's what happened about eighteen months later. Mr. Leibniz had done reasonably well during this interval, although I'd had to increase the dose of his diuretic to keep his legs and abdomen from swelling. One night, with no warning, he had started vomiting blood. By the time the EMS team arrived at his home and got intravenous fluids going, he was unconscious. At the hospital, the emergency room personnel attempted to stabilize him, but they couldn't keep up with the blood loss. He died within hours.

How did so many Americans get the disease? HCV is transmitted by contact with blood or blood products, so risk groups include those who have received blood transfusions, injection drug users, health care workers, and people with exposure to multiple sex partners. Poor people are more likely to have the disease than others. There is no proof that the disease is associated with medical, surgical, or dental procedures or that tattooing, acupuncture, ear piercing, or foreign travel increase the risk. If there is any transmission by these routes, then the frequency may be too low to detect. Age and race are factors too. The 20–40 age range is more likely to be infected than other ranges, Mexican Americans have the disease more frequently than whites, and blacks have the disease more frequently than Mexican Americans. High rates exist among prison inmates—as many as 30 to 40 percent are infected, according to a survey undertaken by the

Rhode Island Department of Corrections in cooperation with the Brown University School of Medicine. Few prison systems test for or treat the disease, so prisons continue to be a large reservoir of infection.

Because donated blood is now screened, and because more sensitive tests have been developed to perform these screenings, the transmission of HCV by blood transfusion has been reduced drastically, though there is still a slight risk of about one in 100,000 units of blood transfused. Immune globulin was at one time a transmitter of HCV, but since December 1994 all immune globulin products must undergo an inactivation procedure or be negative for HCV RNA before release. This has virtually eliminated transmission by this route.

The highest levels of prevalence of HCV infection are found among people who have had frequent repeated percutaneous (through the skin) exposures to blood. This includes injection drug users, people who received blood transfusions from HCV-infected donors, and people with hemophilia who were treated with clotting factor concentrates produced before 1987. There is moderate prevalence among those with smaller direct percutaneous exposure—long-term hemodialysis patients, for example. Still lower prevalence is found among those with less evident percutaneous or with mucosal (through the mucous membranes) exposures—between sex partners, for example—and among those with occasional percutaneous exposures, such as health care workers.

HCV is very efficiently transmitted by the repeated use of contaminated needles—it may even survive the decontamination techniques recommended for HIV—and it has probably been around since the early 1950s. So even someone who hasn't used injection drugs for years can still be a carrier of the disease and can still

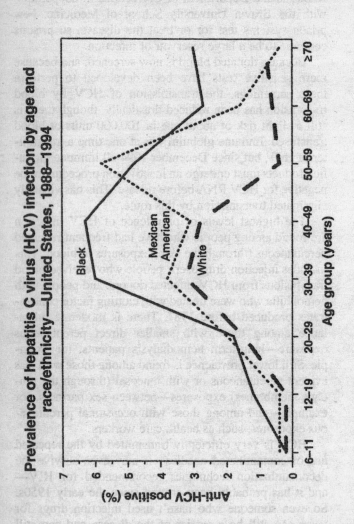

Prevalence of hepatitis C virus (HCV) infection by age and race/ethnicity—United States, 1988–1994

Black

Mexican American

White

Anti-HCV positive (%)

Age group (years)

become ill. While HCV in general is not easy to get, it is easy to get if you come in contact with infected blood—much easier, for example, than HIV. In one drop of blood infected with HIV, there are about 5 virions, or virus particles. In one drop of HCV-infected blood, there are 100,000 virions. This also helps explain why it is very easy for a small amount of HCV-infected blood to contaminate a large blood supply.

It is well-known that HIV can be transmitted by accidental needlesticks, but even among health care workers—those most at risk for this mode of transmission—it may be less well-known that HCV is even easier to transmit this way. The chances of getting HIV from an accidental needlestick are about one in three hundred, but for HCV the chances are one in a hundred. The problem among health care workers may have become more and more evident in recent years because people can be infected with HCV for a long time before they show any symptoms. Some experts believe that cases of HCV infection are now turning up caused by needlesticks or other contacts with blood products that happened before the dangers of such contact were known.

Despite these facts, the number of cases of HCV among injection drug users has declined considerably since 1989, though the incidence (number of new cases) and prevalence (percentage of people in the group who have the infection) are still quite high. HCV is acquired sooner after beginning injections than other viruses. HCV infection among drug users is much higher than HIV infection, and after five years of using injection drugs, 90 percent of people are infected with HCV. This more rapid acquisition of the disease is probably not due to any quality of the virus itself, but rather to the high prevalence of the disease among injection drug users, which increases the chances of exposure.

HCV is also associated with intranasal cocaine use, and some feel this may be because the disease can be transmitted from one nasal membrane to another by shared straws used for sniffing. At the same time, though, among patients with HCV infection, intranasal cocaine use is uncommon in the absence of injection drug use, so it is difficult to say conclusively that intranasal cocaine use is a means of transmission.

HCV can be transmitted in hospitals where infection control techniques are inadequate, but this is extremely rare in the United States except in hemodialysis facilities. Among hemodialysis patients, an average of 10 percent have HCV infection, and there are some centers that report more than half of their patients are infected. The longer a patient has been on dialysis, the more likely he or she is to be infected.

Health care workers are of course at risk from accidental needlestick injuries or other contact with blood. But in fact, HCV infection rates are no higher among health care workers than among the general population—and they are ten times lower than the infection rates for hepatitis B. And this includes orthopedic, general, and oral surgeons, who probably have more exposure to blood than any other health care workers. Even among people who have accidental needlesticks from an HCV-positive source, fewer than 2 percent will get infected. There have been cases of transmission by blood splashes to the eyes, but this is extremely rare.

Patients in hospitals face a very small risk from infected hospital workers. There is one published report of transmission from a cardiothoracic surgeon to five patients in Spain, but the report does not identify what factors contributed to the transmission.

There is an association between sexual activity and the transmission of HCV virus, but some doubt remains about how important sexual contact is in spreading the disease. Certainly any sex practice that involves contact with blood poses some risk. About one-fifth of people infected appear to have no other risk factor except contact with HCV-infected sex partners. Two-thirds of these have a known HCV-infected partner, and the other third have had multiple sex partners in the six-month period preceding the illness. It is probably true of HCV, as it is of other bloodborne viruses, that transmission from men to women is more efficient than transmission from women to men. Whether the sexual contact is homosexual or heterosexual seems to make little difference: the rates of HCV infection among homosexual men are about the same as those of heterosexuals. Rates of infection among the long-term spouses of people with chronic HCV infection are relatively low.

What conclusions can be drawn from the somewhat inconsistent results of studies concerning the sexual transmission of HCV? At this point it is probably fair to say that sexual contact transmits the disease, but not very efficiently. Not enough is known about what other factors may contribute to sexual transmission—kinds of sexual practice engaged in, having another sexually transmitted disease, the viral load of the infectious person, the character of the mucosa of the sexual partners, and so on. In any case, it is probably not quite accurate to classify HCV as an STD.

HCV-positive people with long-term steady partners do not need to change their practices, except insofar as they should discuss their status and the need for testing or counseling with their partner. If your partner tests negative, you will want to understand the available information about transmission by sexual activity and what you can do to prevent spreading the disease. If the partner tests positive, then of course a medical evaluation is required.

How about transmission to nonsexual household contacts? There is certainly an association between HCV infection and infection among household contacts, but the details are still hazy. A toothbrush with blood on it from bleeding gums, a razor blade used by more than one family member, blood on an environmental surface, even a virus contained in other bodily fluids—these are all potential routes of transmission. But no studies so far have managed to eliminate other possible causes of infection besides just living with an infected person. The most accurate conclusion at this point is that household transmission is possible and has almost certainly happened, but it is not common.

About 5 percent of babies born to HCV-infected mothers are themselves infected with the virus, and it doesn't seem to make any difference whether the baby was delivered vaginally or by cesarean section. If the mother has HIV as well as HCV, the rates of transmission of HCV are higher—about 14 percent. Although it isn't absolutely certain that HCV is not transmitted in breast milk, it probably isn't: the rates of infection among breast-fed babies are no different from those among bottle-fed babies.

It is extremely unlikely that HCV can be transmitted by mosquitoes or other insects, and no such case has ever been reported.

About 90 percent of people with HCV have one or more of the risk factors that could explain how they got the disease. But that leaves 10 percent who don't seem to have any of the known risk factors. Most of the people in this 10 percent are poor, and poverty has been associated with many infectious diseases. But preventing HCV among this group is very difficult: If you don't know how they're getting it, how can you tell them what to do to avoid it?

Do You Have It?

Hepatitis C doesn't necessarily have any symptoms, so you can be infected (and potentially infect others) without knowing it until you get some tests. The diagnostic tests are not perfect, and interpreting them can be a challenge.

There are various blood tests that offer information about HCV infection, but only one of them is approved by the U.S. Food and Drug Administration as a diagnostic tool. This test, called an ELISA, or enzyme linked immunosorbent assay, detects the presence of anti-HCV in the blood—not the virus itself, but the antibody that the immune system creates to fight it. It takes as long as two months after infection for the test to come up with a positive result. This test doesn't tell you whether you have an acute infection, a chronic infection, or an infection that has gone away completely—it only tells you if you have the antibodies in your blood. The test went through two previous versions before the one that is used today, called ELISA III, was developed.

ELISA III is not an expensive test, and is often used as the first step in testing for HCV. But even though ELISA III is more accurate than earlier versions, false-positive results are still common in populations where the disease is rare. So if you get a positive result on this test—that is, if the test indicates the presence of the antibody—then you need a supplemental test to be sure there isn't a mistake. The supplemental test, performed on a blood sample that has come out positive for the initial test, is called the recombinant immunoblot assay, or RIBA. This too is now available in a third-generation version.

With this supplemental test there are three possible results: negative, positive, or indeterminate. If you get a positive result on this test, you are infected with HCV. If you get a negative result on the RIBA, you are considered uninfected unless there is some other reason to believe you are infected (for example, if you have liver disease with no other explanation for it). And finally—nothing is simple here—you can get an indeterminate result, which might indicate that you are actually not infected, or might suggest that you are in the early stages of an HCV infection and have not yet "seroconverted," that is, shown evidence of the production of antibodies in your blood.

More Tests

What we've described above is the standard procedure. But there are other tests, not yet approved for use in diagnosis by the FDA (not because they are dangerous—they aren't—but because their reliability and accuracy are insufficient or still in question). One other way to detect the presence of HCV infection is to look for the ribonucleic acid (RNA) that is characteristic of the virus. This can be found using a technique called gene amplification, and the test will work within about one to two weeks after exposure to the virus. The test's name is a mouthful: the reverse transcriptase polymerase chain reaction amplification of HCV RNA, or RT-PCR for short. This is also called the test for "viral load."

The sample has to be handled very carefully for the test to work at all. You can't just take some blood, stick it in a test tube, and do the test. The serum has to be separated from cellular components within four hours of collection, and stored frozen between -20 and $-70°C$. The sample has to be kept frozen until the test can be performed, and rigorous quality control is essential in any lab attempting the test. The results don't produce a simple yes or no, because not everyone who is infected will test positive for this assay. But the large majority of infected people will. The test is quite expensive to perform, and is not routinely offered in most settings.

The RT-PCR test indicates the presence of HCV RNA, but doesn't reveal how concentrated it is in the blood sample. For this, there are other tests that can be performed. One is called the Amplicor HCV Monitor; another is the Quantiplex HCV RNA Assay. These two tests, manufactured by two different companies, use different standards, so it's hard to compare them. While knowing the concentration of HCV RNA in the blood might predict how well a patient would respond to antiviral therapy, these tests have not yet proven useful in clinical practice. For now they are used only in doing research.

Liver Function Tests

Liver function tests won't tell you anything about the presence or absence of HCV, but they can determine if the liver is functioning normally. They do this by testing various biochemical indicators. Alanine aminotransferase (ALT) and aspartate aminotransferase (AST) are the two most common. These enzymes, normally present inside liver cells, leak into the bloodstream when the cells are

Hepatitus C virus (HCV) infection testing algorithm for asymptomatic persons

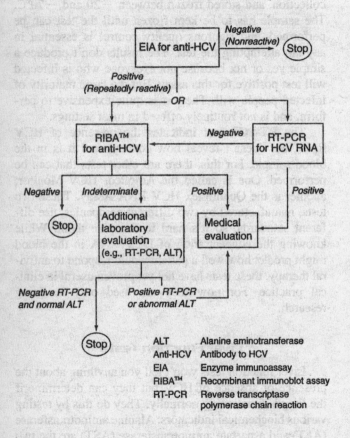

ALT	Alanine aminotransferase
Anti-HCV	Antibody to HCV
EIA	Enzyme immunoassay
RIBA™	Recombinant immunoblot assay
RT-PCR	Reverse transcriptase polymerase chain reaction

damaged, so if they are found in the blood in excessive quantities, there is a problem with the liver. Alkaline phosphate levels may increase with bad liver functioning, and there is a test for the presence of this enzyme. There are also tests for bilirubin levels, to suggest the state of the bile duct and the liver's efficiency in clearing the blood of the substances formed when hemoglobin is broken down; for albumin, to determine how well the liver is forming protein; for prothrombin, to tell how well the liver is producing the substance that helps clot blood; and for caffeine clearance, because clearing caffeine from the blood is one of the liver's functions, and slow clearing of caffeine may mean a malfunctioning liver. And there are more tests for other substances in the blood; these are under development and their significance is still not known, or not fully understood.

Ultrasound and CAT Scans

Ultrasound tests can reveal an irregular surface on the liver, which usually indicates cirrhosis, and they can also detect lymph node abnormalities. CAT (computer assisted tomography) scans, which are quite expensive, can also reveal some information. Cirrhotic livers are usually small. Fatty livers are more homogeneous and are enlarged. Both tests are used to determine if gallstones are present and if there is any obstruction and/or dilation of the bile ducts. These give information about the anatomy of the entire liver. A biopsy (discussed below) gives information at the cellular level.

Biopsy

Because blood tests don't give a complete picture of the health of the liver, probably the only fully reliable way of determining the presence of an HCV infection is by taking a biopsy of the liver. In this procedure, a thin needle is inserted into the liver and a sample of tissue is removed and then examined under a microscope to determine the extent of liver injury.

A liver biopsy is not a terribly risky procedure; nor is it particularly pleasant. The most dangerous complication is bleeding, and patients usually have to stay in the hospital, lying as still as possible for about six hours after the procedure, to make sure this doesn't happen. Usually only local anesthetic is used during the procedure, along with Valium or other tranquilizers. Patients report varying degrees of discomfort. Sometimes pain in the right shoulder makes it difficult for the patient to lie still after the procedure, and the pain may be severe enough to require opiates.

Biopsy results are usually reported as a "stage" indicating the amount of inflammation. The stages are numbered from 0 to 6, with 0 indicating no disease and 6 indicating cirrhosis of the liver. In many cases, biopsy is the only certain way to determine the extent of disease and the kind of treatment that should be undertaken.

Who Should Be Tested for HCV?

The CDC doesn't recommend that everyone be tested for HCV—the disease isn't so common that universal testing is necessary or desirable. Anyone who is concerned about his or her HCV status should of course follow through with tests, but in general the CDC recommends that testing should be routinely done only among people who are in certain specific risk groups, and among those who have had a known exposure to HCV-positive blood.

- Anyone who has ever injected illegal drugs—even if only once or many years ago—should be tested. Since people who inject illegal drugs may not be seen in ordinary health care settings, the CDC urges community-based organizations to seek these people out for testing, counseling, and medical follow-up. The exact methods of outreach that would be best for this population are still not known, and further study is required.
- People with hemophilia who received clotting factor concentrates before 1987, as well as long-term hemodialysis patients, should be tested, as should anyone who received a blood transfusion or organ transplant before July 1992 (when routine screening of blood for HCV was instituted).
- Sometimes people who get liver function tests for other reasons will have abnormally high levels of ALT (alanine aminotransferase) or AST (aspartate aminotransferase), the enzymes (discussed above) that may appear in the blood when the liver isn't functioning properly. This elevation alone doesn't mean you have HCV, but you should be tested for HCV if these readings are persistently above normal.

Some Implications of Testing for HCV

Some people may be hesitant to find out what their HCV status is, and with good reason, since the disease is often stigmatized. Employers may be negatively influenced by such a diagnosis. Health insurance may be more difficult or more expensive to obtain. Children may be discriminated against if it is learned that their parents are infected. Doctors may assume that if you have hepatitis

C, you must be an injection drug user. Even friends and family can have unpredictable reactions. Issues of stigma are real, and must be balanced against the potential seriousness of the disease and the existence of efficacious treatment.

In May 1999 the FDA approved an over-the-counter testing kit for hepatitis C antibodies. This kit, called Hepatitis C Check, is manufactured by Home Access Health Company of Estates, Illinois. It contains a lancet for getting a drop of blood, filter paper, and a mailer. The patient takes a sample of his own blood, then mails it to a laboratory for analysis. The kit has a unique personal identification number so that the results can be obtained anonymously.

The procedures of requiring informed consent and post-test counseling that have been instituted for HIV testing are usually not applied to HCV testing, although they probably should be. There are facilities where you can be tested anonymously, but if you are positive, and if you want a complete set of tests, it will be almost impossible to get them without revealing that you are an HCV patient. In general, informed consent should be given for HCV testing just as for other medical procedures, and measures should be taken to prevent unwanted disclosure of the results of the test.

When you are tested for HCV, you should be provided with complete information about:

- What kind of exposure might have caused you to get HCV
- The test procedures and the meaning of test results
- The health benefits of early detection
- Available medical treatments
- The potential risks of testing positive, including

disrupted personal relationships, the possibility of job discrimination, the risk of loss of employment, the effect on health insurance, and the possible effect on educational opportunities
- For those who test positive, information about transmission both to adults and children

Wherever the test is performed—and it can be done in a physician's office, a health department clinic, or another health care facility—such facilities must be prepared to provide the appropriate information about the disease, as well as referral, if necessary, to additional medical care, substance abuse services, and support groups.

5

Hepatitis C

TREATMENT, AND THE
POSSIBILITY OF A CURE

You now know the symptoms of hepatitis C. You
know if you're in one of the risk groups. You know
what tests are available and what they mean. So you
know if you should visit a doctor and get a diagnosis.
But this may not be as straightforward a procedure as you
think. Hepatitis C is not a routine or easy diagnosis, and
not all doctors are capable of making it. In fact, of the
30,000 new cases of HCV every year, only about a third
are diagnosed. Many of the symptoms of HCV are
vague—tiredness, malaise, mental cloudiness—and
many doctors will believe, correctly, that these can be the
symptoms of many diseases, or of no disease at all. So it
may not be easy to convince a doctor—or for a doctor to
convince him- or herself—that a disease as serious as
hepatitis C is the cause. A referral to a specialist may be
required, and it may be that you, armed with the facts
about hepatitis C, will have to be the one to take matters
into your own hands and demand a referral to a gastroenterologist, preferably to a hepatologist (liver specialist).

This referral can come from your general practitioner or internist, or you may use one or more of the organizations listed in the resources section of this book. Many HCV patients are treated for long periods of time for secondary symptoms, or not treated at all, before the correct diagnosis is made. You can avoid this by getting the diagnosis right in the first place.

If you still think that a specialist isn't really necessary, and that your ordinary family doctor can take care of you as well as anyone, a recent survey of 404 primary care physicians may give you cause to wonder. Twenty percent still believed that blood transfusion was a significant risk factor for HCV infection (which it has not been since blood screening procedures were initiated in the early 1990s), and 33 percent would follow a hepatitis C patient by themselves even though none of them had ever treated one before. Almost a third didn't know the efficacy of interferon treatment. None of this should inspire confidence in the ability of general practitioners to treat hepatitis C effectively.

You've had the tests, you've had a biopsy, you've been to the specialists, and they've given you the bad news: you have hepatitis C. Now what? There are specific things you can do to improve how you feel—and maybe even find a cure. There are essentially three choices for HCV patients, depending on the nature of the infection and the amount of liver damage it is causing: (1) no treatment at all, (2) antiviral drug therapy, and (3) liver transplant. But no matter what treatment regimen you and your doctor decide to follow, there are certain essential lifestyle changes you must make.

The clinical course of hepatitis C is poorly understood, largely because the onset of the illness so often goes unrecognized. Except in cases where the patient has had transfusions or been the victim of an accidental needlestick, it is almost impossible to specify exactly when an infection began. To add to the problem, there are many subtypes of the virus, geographical differences in types of infection, varying dietary habits (particularly as concerns alcohol consumption), and any number of other unexplained factors, all of which may or may not influence the course of the illness.

There are, nevertheless, certain generalizations that can be made. HCV RNA can be detected in the blood of an infected person within about three weeks of the infection. Within two months of this time, almost all infected people have suffered some liver damage, and this is reflected in high readings of serum alanine aminotransferase (ALT) in their blood samples. Still, despite whatever liver damage is being done at this point, most patients don't have any symptoms—they don't get the flulike symptoms characteristic of hepatitis A or B, and they don't become jaundiced. Both hepatitis A and hepatitis B can lead to fulminant infections that can be fatal, but this almost never happens with hepatitis C. Instead, hepatitis C usually becomes a chronic infection. About 15 percent of patients clear the virus from their blood within six months, and their liver function tests return to normal. The rest become chronic hepatitis C carriers.

This chronic disease has a variable course, but most patients suffer no symptoms at all during the first two decades after infection. Some experience intermittent fatigue, malaise, or other nonspecific discomforts. More often the first real symptom of the illness is advanced liver disease. The virus makes liver cells inflamed, and these inflamed cells begin to enter the portal tracts (the place under the liver where the liver's ducts are located), sometimes collecting in small numbers at the edges of the organ near the ducts. As more and more cells are involved, fibrosis begins—essentially, scar tissue begins to form on the liver. This is the beginning of cirrhosis, the destruction of the liver by repeated inflammation and scarring of tissue.

If you have HCV, an infection with hepatitis A or hepatitis B can be deadly. Even though HBV DNA seems to inhibit HCV RNA replication, patients infected with both viruses generally have more severe liver disease than those with only one. Hepatocellular carcinoma—liver cancer—is more common in people with both infections than in those with HCV alone. Fortunately, there are vaccines for both hepatitis A and hepatitis B, and anyone with HCV should have those vaccines. HCV-infected people with concurrent HIV infection and good clinical status should be treated for HCV, because they are likely to have an accelerated course of disease.

There is at least one case report of a hepatitis C patient superinfected with hepatitis B whose hepatitis C seemed to clear completely after the hepatitis B infection passed. With the appearance of an acute hepatitis B infection, serum hepatitis C virus RNA became undetectable. At the same time, there was a significant increase in the antibodies to hepatitis C. The acute hepatitis B infection then passed, and hepatitis B surface antigen was undetectable. Within two years, hepatitis C virus RNA was also undetectable. The authors of the case report hypothesize that the acute hepatitis B infection stimulated response against hepatitis C as well, eventually eliminating both viruses. Despite this, no one would recommend infection with hepatitis B as a means of curing hepatitis C.

About one-fifth of HCV-infected patients will develop cirrhosis within twenty years of infection, and the progression is considerably faster if you drink alcohol. So one of the first things anyone with a diagnosis of hepatitis C will have to do is to stop using alcohol completely. If you are using injection drugs or drinking more than one alcoholic drink a day, you will not be eligible for anti-HCV therapy until six months after these practices are stopped.

Although the risk of transmitting hepatitis C during sexual contact is low, the surest way to avoid contracting any sexually transmitted disease is to have sex with only one uninfected partner or not to have sex at all. If you already have HCV, there is a low, but real, danger of transmitting it to your uninfected partner. Using latex condoms during sex is essential.

Since anyone who touches your blood is at some risk, you should inform any health care workers with whom you come in contact of your HCV status. At the same time, health care workers should be taking universal precautions—that is, protecting themselves from contact with anyone's blood, under the assumption that anyone can be infected.

Difficult Treatment, Successful Outcome

Charlie Mistretta was coming in for an initial visit. He was a good-looking man who appeared to be in his late thirties, stocky and well-muscled. As we shook hands, I noticed that the letters *h*, *a*, *t*, and *e* were crudely tattooed on the second through fifth fingers.

He caught my downward glance and laughed. "I had a wild youth, and that's a memento from a prison I spent some time in. I think there were a few years I hated everybody, myself most of all. Fortunately, that was a while ago now."

Charlie had grown up on the streets of a rough neighborhood. He didn't have much to say about his parents, and it was clear that he had been on his own from an early age. He started smoking marijuana and drinking cheap wine at age twelve; by sixteen, he was shooting heroin. He was in and out of substance abuse programs and prison for more than ten years, but then something clicked for him, and he used a twelve-month inpatient drug program to convince himself that he wanted to be clean. That was almost ten years ago, and now he was married with one child and working as a substance abuse counselor.

He remembered having one serious illness: subacute bacterial endocarditis, an infection of the heart valves. He had been gravely ill and had received six weeks of intravenous antibiotics. Other than that, he had been fine except for several cases of gonorrhea. He was feeling fine now, but wanted a thorough checkup.

His physical exam was remarkable only for a soft heart murmur that presumably came from scarring of one of the heart valves. We talked about HIV, and he agreed to be tested. He knew that he should have been tested years ago, and he clearly felt guilty about possibly having exposed his wife and child to the virus.

His HIV test was negative, but his liver serologies were filled with positives. The hepatitis A IgG was positive, indicating an old infection; his anti-HBs (hepatitis B surface antibody) and anti-HBc (hepatitis B core antibody) tests were positive—another old infection that had been cleared from the body. Unfortunately, the hepatitis C antibody test was also positive, and that almost always indicates active disease. The fact that his AST and ALT were more than twice normal suggested active disease as well. All his other tests were fine.

He had a worried look when he walked into my office to get the test results. Most people worry the most about HIV, and I quickly assured him that the test was

negative. He visibly relaxed. I then told him about the
hepatitis C, explaining that there was no evidence of serious damage to his liver at this time, but letting him
know that the potential for it definitely existed. His first
question was whether his wife and child might have it. I
explained that sexual transmission was possible but not
likely, and it might be best for his wife to be tested. As
for his child, the chances were even slimmer, since only
a small percentage of babies born to hepatitis C positive
women are infected at birth. There was no point in testing his child until after his wife was tested.

I told him I wanted to do some more sophisticated
tests before discussing treatment, and he agreed. It
seemed that he had heard enough for one day.

I drew an RT-PCR (viral load) test and a hepatitis C
genotype. The viral load was about 1,000,000, and I
quickly explained to Charlie that it wasn't as bad as it
sounded. In fact, anything less than 2,000,000 was generally considered to increase the likelihood of a positive
response to treatment. The fact that he had genotype 1
hepatitis C, however, was not a good prognostic sign,
since type 1 virus is less likely to respond to treatment
and usually requires a longer period on the combination
of interferon and ribavirin.

Charlie and I discussed his treatment options at some
length when he returned for his third visit. We also discussed the possibility of a liver biopsy, but he said there
was no way he was getting a needle stuck in his liver. He
wanted to be aggressive and treat the infection, and I
assured him we could do that without the biopsy.

I told him about some of the most common and unpleasant side effects associated with both interferon and
ribavirin and warned him that treatment would probably
last a full year. The odds of success—success being defined by normalization of liver enzymes and the RT-PCR
test becoming negative—were about fifty-fifty. I told him

that he and his wife would have to use two forms of birth control while he was taking the ribavirin because it was known to cause severe birth defects. I told him there was no emergency and that he should take his time thinking it over and discuss it with his wife. He left with several pamphlets about hepatitis C and its treatment.

He returned a month later, ready to start treatment. I explained that interferon was traditionally given three times a week, but that I was increasingly convinced that taking smaller doses every day was more likely to work. He agreed to that regimen, promising that he and his wife were using condoms and birth control pills.

Charlie got through the first month of treatment better than almost any patient I had seen. By month two, however, he complained of feeling depressed, finding little pleasure at home or at work. He found himself teary, and was getting up at 4 A.M. I reminded him about depression being a potential side effect of interferon, and he said that something had to be done or else he would stop the treatment. It was ruining his life.

I told him that I thought he should reduce the dose of interferon for now, and I suggested that he start an antidepressant. He agreed to both changes and said he'd come back in two weeks. I told him to call if he was feeling worse instead of better.

I didn't hear from him during those two weeks, and he clearly looked more like his old self when he walked into my office. He said he was still having some minor side effects from the interferon but that the depression was largely gone. He felt ready to continue the treatment. Charlie finished the twelve-month course, although he required injections for anemia caused by the ribavirin. His RT-PCR is now negative, and he will need to have it checked every six months.

Who Should Be Treated?

The treatments for HCV infection are expensive, only sometimes efficacious, and carry many risks, so not everyone with HCV infection is a candidate for treatment. While with certain groups of patients treatment is clearly recommended, with others the decision to begin treatment is not so clear, and decisions must be made on a case-by-case basis.

Patients at the greatest risk for developing cirrhosis should certainly be treated. Who are these people? Anyone who is HCV-infected, has persistently high ALT levels, is positive for HCV RNA, and whose liver biopsy shows moderate degrees of inflammation and necrosis. These people are in danger of getting a fatal illness—cirrhosis or liver cancer—and must be treated.

With others, however, the decision isn't so clear. Some people with elevated ALT levels have nevertheless suffered little in the way of liver damage, and may not suffer any liver dysfunction for years, if ever. Treating such patients with antiviral therapy is not recommended. Instead, their levels of ALT should be monitored and a liver biopsy performed every three to five years. Interferon treatment for patients with normal ALT is not beneficial—in fact, it may be harmful in that it can actually cause abnormalities in liver enzyme production.

Race is a factor not only in the prevalence of hepatitis C (see chapter 4), but apparently also in the response to treatment. Authors of a recent study found that African American patients do not respond as well to treatment with interferon as Hispanics, Asian Americans, and non-Hispanic white patients. No one knows why this should be so. The differences in virological response were significant enough that the authors of the study believe they should be considered both in assessing trials of interferon therapy and in counseling patients about treatment.

Some patients have "compensated cirrhosis"—some liver damage, but no jaundice, no accumulation of fluid in the abdominal cavity, no damage to the veins leading to the liver, and no evidence of brain involvement. There is no evidence that antiviral therapy improves the survival chances of such patients, so they should not be treated either. Similarly, there is not yet any proof that antiviral therapy helps people under eighteen or over sixty, so decisions on the treatment of any of these groups should be made on an individual basis after a thorough discussion and complete understanding on the part of the patient of the risks and benefits of undergoing therapy. Moreover—and this is important—the National Institutes of Health urges that if therapy is undertaken with these patients, it be done in the context of clinical trials so that data can be collected for future decision making.

Who Should Not Be Treated?

Current medicines for HCV are not highly effective, and they have many serious side effects. People who drink heavily cannot be treated, because alcohol directly interferes with the antiviral effects of interferon and ribavirin. People who are using drugs cannot be treated, because they risk reinfecting themselves. In addition, people who drink heavily or use drugs are unlikely to be compliant with the rather complex procedures required for effective treatment. And finally, people who already have serious liver damage cannot be treated, because the treatment may make them sicker. Whether patients with mild liver disease should be treated is still a matter of some controversy, as is treating older people with other serious disorders.

Not Everyone Wants Treatment—
At Least Not Right Now

Josh Borden was in his early forties but looked younger. That was probably due to his ponytail and fashionably stubbled beard. His handshake was strong and I noticed the grease around his nails, which went along with his being a car mechanic. The insurance company for the car dealership he worked for had referred him for evaluation after he tested positive for hepatitis C.

He started talking before we even had a chance to sit down.

"Doc, I don't know what the big deal is. I feel great. I've got no problem talking to you, but I want you to know that I've never felt better."

"Mr. Borden, that's great. Feeling well makes everything easier. But if it's okay, I'd just like to explain some of your test results to you and see if you have any questions."

"No problem. Go ahead, Doc."

"As you know, you had several blood tests when you had your insurance physical. Most of your tests and your electrocardiogram were perfect. There were two tests involving your liver that weren't quite normal. One of them we call a liver function test, and that showed that there's some inflammation in your liver; those numbers were about three times as high as they should be. The other was a test for a kind of virus called hepatitis C that can cause liver disease. That was positive also."

"Is that bad, Doc?"

"Well, not necessarily, but they could cause you problems down the line. First, of all, let me ask you a few questions that might help explain how you got the hepatitis C virus."

Mr. Borden, it turned out, had never injected drugs, but had sniffed cocaine with friends over the years. Perhaps most important, he had had a motorcycle accident in his mid-twenties and had required multiple transfusions.

"Well, the most likely cause for the hepatitis were those transfusions you got in 1986. But we still don't know if it's the hepatitis C virus that's causing those liver function abnormalities. Let me ask you about some other things that might affect your liver."

Mr. Borden said that he didn't have much exposure to chemicals on the job, and he denied taking any medications, even Tylenol or aspirin, regularly. He did, however, like to drink beer.

"Josh, when you say you like to drink beer, do you mean you drink it every day?"

"Well, more or less."

"How many cans a day?"

"Not that many."

"Tell me what you had to drink yesterday."

"Yesterday? I probably had one or two cans—two cans, actually—with lunch. Then I went out with some of the guys right after work and had a couple at the bar. I had one or two with supper at home. Probably seven or eight altogether."

Josh said that some days were more than that and some days were less.

"Josh, it may be that the beer itself is causing your liver tests to go up. Whether it's the beer or the hepatitis C, the combination isn't good for your liver. And, if we're ever going to treat the hepatitis C, you're going to need to really cut back on the alcohol or, better yet, cut it out completely. You can't take the medicines for hepatitis C and continue to drink like that."

"Doc, I hear what you're saying, but I like my beer. It relaxes me . . . smoothes out any problems I have at the job or at home. You understand?"

"Yes, I do understand. But it may be really damaging your liver. It's my job to make sure you understand that. Do you understand? I can refer you to a program that will help you get some control over the drinking."

"Doc, I really appreciate that, but I just can't handle that right now. You sure there's nothing you can just give me for the hepatitis C?"

"Josh, I would if I could. But the treatment for hepatitis C involves taking shots and pills for a year. And they won't work if you're drinking. Think about it, and if you want to talk more about it, just call for another appointment."

"Absolutely, Doc. I'll let you know when I'm ready. Pleasure to meet you."

Beginning Treatment

Although there are good diagnostic tests for the presence of HCV, they are not very useful for monitoring the progress of the disease once you have it. Levels of the ALT enzyme in the blood—the most common test—can vary considerably during the course of the disease, and they reveal little or nothing about the actual condition of the liver. Still, the ALT, and the test for AST, are useful for measuring the effectiveness of antiviral therapy.

Similarly, testing for HCV RNA by reverse transcriptase polymerase chain reaction (RT-PCR), while not useful for monitoring the progression of illness, is a fairly accurate measure of the success of antiviral therapy. This test, sometimes called a test of "viral load," can also predict response to interferon. In addition, successful treatment correlates with a low viral load at the outset.

The most accurate measure of progress is liver biopsy, and, although there is now some question about its benefits for treatment outcome, most doctors will want you to have a liver biopsy before treatment begins. This will give an accurate picture of the severity of your illness and the degree of liver damage you're suffering. It is also used to exclude other forms of liver disease besides hepatitis C, and to assess what damage may be caused by alcohol use, other medications, or excess iron that has been deposited in the liver. This test is expensive and uncomfortable and carries at least some risk (see chapter 4 for details), but you may nevertheless need periodic biopsies during the course of your illness. At the same time, more and more doctors now believe that the biopsy may not be necessary to decide if treatment has been successful—they consider the normalization of ALT and the absence of HCV RNA a good indication that treatment has worked. Clinicians will repeat these tests every six months for several years to make sure things are still going well.

Interferon for Hepatitis C

Interferons are small protein molecules that the body secretes in response to viral infections. There are two major groups of these proteins, called type I and type II, and many subtypes within each large group. They do their work of combating viruses by attaching themselves to receptors on the cell surface. Once attached, they cause a complex sequence of events inside the cell that includes the production of certain enzymes. Biologists believe that these enzymes cause the virus to stop replicating inside the cell, generating the therapeutic effect.

Interferon can be manufactured using recombinant

gene technology. The technique is extremely complex, with many carefully regulated steps, but at the heart of the process is the genetic alteration of a cell by the insertion of a synthetically constructed genetic sequence that codes for the protein. The cells used are often bacteria—*E. coli,* one of the bacteria that lives in the intestines of healthy people, is used by some manufacturers.

As with hepatitis B, interferon is the drug approved for treating hepatitis C. With subcutaneous injections of interferon three times a week for one year, about 50 percent of hepatitis C patients have normal serum ALT activity, and 33 percent have no detectable HCV RNA in their blood. But when therapy is stopped, about half these patients relapse. So roughly 15 percent to 25 percent of patients treated with interferon have a sustained response from taking the drug as measured by ALT readings one year after therapy ends. If you take interferon for three months without any reduction in your ALT levels or change in detectable HCV RNA, the medicine probably won't help you. Interferon has been shown to be less effective in patients with higher HCV RNA levels and in patients with HCV genotype 1. Unfortunately, genotype 1 is the most common strain in the United States. But neither high HCV RNA nor having genotype 1 is a reason to avoid interferon therapy.

As we noted in chapter 3, interferon is not an easy medicine to use. First, you must have a doctor with experience in using the medicine—a general practitioner is unlikely to have the required expertise. When using interferon for hepatitis C, you have to inject it (in smaller doses than for treating hepatitis B), usually several times a week. The injection can be either subcutaneous (under the skin) or intramuscular (into a muscle), but there is no available pill, because stomach acid destroys interferon.

The proper places to inject the medicine are the upper arm, the thigh, or the abdomen. There is a pill form of alpha interferon under development, but it is still experimental, and a Canadian company announced in June 1999 that they had had success with a skin-patch form of interferon that delivers the medicine through the skin without an injection. This form is not now approved for use in treating hepatitis.

Since the injections are so frequent over such a long period of time, the only practical way to administer them is to do it yourself. This means you have to learn how to inject yourself using a disposable syringe, and you have to carefully follow all directions given by your doctor and in the patient instruction sheet given with the medicine. You will have to consult with a doctor or pharmacist about the safest way to dispose of used syringes. The medicine has to be refrigerated, but not frozen. You have to examine the medicine for discoloration or particulate matter before you inject it, and discard it if it's discolored or if there is stuff floating in it.

Interferon doesn't work for everyone, and, when it does work, how well it works depends on the patient. After three months of treatment, you will get another blood test to see if it is doing what it should. At this point a decision has to be made about whether to continue therapy. If there is little change in your blood test, the doctor will probably advise stopping therapy at this point. But this is an individual judgment that can only be made after careful discussion with your doctor.

If the medicine is having its intended effect after the first three months, the therapy will continue for six to twelve months. Again, there is considerable variation from patient to patient when considering how long therapy should continue, and you will have to consult with your physician.

Combination Therapy with Ribavirin

Interferon, obviously, doesn't work as well as we'd like. Only about 15 percent of hepatitis C patients who take it have a cure—in the sense that they don't relapse after they finish the course of medicine. For some time, however, doctors have noticed that if they administer another drug along with interferon, an antiviral drug called ribavirin, the combination works much better than interferon alone.

Ribavirin is one of the first antiviral drugs ever discovered, so doctors have had considerable experience in using it. When used by itself, unlike interferon, it doesn't have many serious side effects. It has been used for some time for the treatment of severe lung infections in infants.

A study published in the *New England Journal of Medicine* in the fall of 1998 confirmed the clinical observation that interferon and ribavirin together work better than interferon alone. The study considered both the effects of initial treatment and the problem of relapse. At the end of six months of treatment, about half the patients who took interferon alone had undetectable levels of HCV RNA, but about 82 percent of the patients on combination therapy had those undetectable levels. Six months after cessation of treatment, only 5 percent of those using interferon alone had undetectable levels of HCV RNA, while 49 percent of patients using the combination therapy had undetectable levels. Other studies, including large clinical trials, confirmed these results. In June 1999 the FDA approved the combination use of ribavirin capsules and interferon injections for the treatment of hepatitis C.

The combination therapy is more effective, but it also has more side effects, and some people cannot tolerate them. In the study cited above, the authors reported that drug doses had to be reduced or treatment discontinued more often with the combination therapy than with the interferon alone.

Ribavirin by itself doesn't have any effect on the hepatitis C virus. But it appears to help interferon do its work in strengthening the immune system.

This combination treatment requires three subcutaneous injections of interferon per week, plus 1,000 to 1,200 milligrams of ribavirin (depending on the weight of the patient) taken in divided daily doses, morning and evening, for twenty-four weeks. Schering-Plough packages their brands of interferon (Intron) and ribavirin (Rebetol) together as Rebetron combination therapy. There are several companies that manufacture interferon, but until its license ran out in 1999 only Schering-Plough made ribavirin. The drug is now becoming available from other sources.

How long should you take these medicines? This is a complex question, still not completely settled, but current practice dictates that it depends on the kind of HCV you are infected with. Six months of treatment is recommended for patients with genotype 2 or 3, regardless of the viral load. For genotype 1, the most common in North America, six months is enough if viral load is low, but twelve months may be required if it is not. The combination of interferon and ribavirin given for a year eliminates the virus in about 40 percent of patients.

Side Effects of Interferon

As we noted in our discussion of hepatitis B, interferon has many side effects, and some are quite unpleasant. Among the most common are mild to moderate flulike symptoms—fever, muscle aches, chills, and fatigue. Some people will feel irritable or depressed (although these may be symptoms of hepatitis C itself). Partial hair loss, irregular heartbeat, and numbness in the fingers, toes, and face can also occur.

Some of the drug's worst side effects are psychiatric. If you have a history of depression, interferon is a particularly difficult drug to use. It can cause depression so severe that it leads to suicidal ideation and suicide attempts. If this happens, the drug should be stopped. If you are on interferon and begin to feel depressed, you must report it to your physician immediately. Nervousness, emotional lability, abnormal thinking, agitation, and apathy are other adverse psychiatric events that interferon can cause. Antidepressants can be used for the side effects of interferon, but they can be poisonous to the liver, so they have to be monitored extremely carefully.

No one who has severe hepatic disease should be using interferon, and if you develop symptoms of liver decompensation—jaundice, decreased serum albumin, fluid accumulation in the abdomen, and so on—you should stop taking interferon. People with autoimmune diseases should not use interferon; those with cardiac problems must be watched very carefully, as should anyone with endocrine disorders. Pregnant women should not use interferon, and no one knows if interferon is excreted in breast milk, or, if it is, whether it harms a baby or not.

The most common side effect—the flulike symptoms—can be treated with Tylenol or other nonnarcotic analgesics. (While Tylenol can be bad for the liver, it's all a matter of quantity: less than 4 grams per day—eight 500 mg tablets in 24 hours—is quite safe. Aspirin and other nonsteroidal anti-inflammatory drugs—Motrin or Advil, for example—can be worse.) Taking the interferon shots at night before you go to bed also helps, as then you can sleep through the worst of the side effects. Some people on interferon have taken ibuprofen for the joint pain, but this is not a good idea. In some recent case reports, ibuprofen has caused a significant increase in liver enzymes in the blood, even in low doses, and this suggests that the ibuprofen is causing liver damage.

You shouldn't give up on the medicine because of side effects—in fact, they may be proof that it's working. But you should keep your doctor informed about whatever side effects you are feeling. Usually they lessen as treatment continues, and some people don't experience them at all.

Side Effects and Precautions with Ribavirin

Ribavirin is approved by the FDA for only two uses: very severe lung infections in newborns, and combination therapy for HCV. But it is widely used for treating influenza A and other diseases, including HIV. Ribavirin can cause hemolytic anemia, intolerance to cold, and shortness of breath, as well as irregular heartbeats, lung malfunctions, and hypotension.

If you have asthma or heart problems, you shouldn't use ribavirin. And if you are pregnant, nursing, or even planning to get pregnant, you shouldn't use it. In fact, in February 1999, six months after the FDA approved ribavirin and interferon combination for initial HCV therapy,

Schering-Plough issued a new warning that patients and their sexual partners must use two forms of contraception because of the risk of birth defects or loss of a pregnancy, even if only one of the partners is on the therapy. And don't be surprised if the doctor asks you to put this agreement in writing. If you aren't willing or able to practice this kind of contraception, you should not be using ribavirin. People with kidney disease cannot tolerate ribavirin, nor can those with severe heart disease. Its use in older people or those with arterial hypertension must be undertaken with great care.

Some of these side effects can persist for months after stopping therapy. All this makes deciding to use the drug a complex problem that must be decided on a case-by-case basis. It is not for everyone.

Current Practice

An article published in August 1999 in the *Journal of the American Medical Association* summarizes current practice in the treatment of chronic hepatitis C. In general, a candidate for treatment will have a persistently elevated ALT, and a viral load test that indicates the presence of circulating HCV RNA. The treatment of patients who have normal ALT levels is still controversial. Liver biopsies, widely recommended before beginning treatment, do not actually increase the success of the treatment, although they do increase the cost. It is now believed that a better approach may be to do liver biopsies only for people who do not respond to treatment. Your viral load is not a factor in deciding to go ahead with treatment, but it does predict how long the treatment with interferon and ribavirin will take.

Using interferon alone three times weekly for a year

results in only about 20 percent of patients getting better, but larger and more frequent doses are now being studied for efficacy. Often, if a patient doesn't get better after a year of treatment—that is, fails to clear HCV RNA from his blood—therapy will be stopped. But some now believe that continued therapy even after a year may be valuable for slowing the progression of the disease, even if HCV RNA is still present.

Combination therapy with ribavirin and interferon, while it is not a miracle cure, does improve results—about 38 percent of patients improve on the combination. Probably the ribavirin acts as an antiviral agent while the interferon modifies the immune system and reduces inflammation. Genotype 1 patients respond more poorly than others.

Liver Transplantation

If liver damage is so great that the liver can no longer function, the only treatment left is liver transplantation. This is of course a difficult operation, fraught with complex problems, from the acquisition of a suitable organ through the maintenance of health after the operation. Liver transplantation has been performed since 1963, and has been perfected over the years. Today about 80 percent of liver transplants result in survival for more than five years.

One of the many problems in transplanting a liver into an HCV patient is that the new liver can, and usually does, become infected with HCV. Sometimes this new liver disease progresses so slowly that it doesn't matter, but in other cases the new organ is rapidly damaged. This may be because of the use of immunosuppressants to prevent the rejection of the foreign organ.

Healthy livers for transplant are in seriously short supply, but researchers have found that hepatitis C infected livers may be an option for people who are already infected. Infected livers had been routinely considered unfit for transplant, but doctors now believe that survival rates with infected livers are not significantly different from survival rates with healthy livers. The researchers found that the best results were obtained when infected patients received a liver infected with a different strain of the virus from the one they had. The new strain does not cause significant disease in the new liver even if it becomes predominant in the blood. In cases where an uninfected liver is transplanted, reinfection of the new liver is almost inevitable.

Recently, attempts have been made to transplant part of a liver from a living donor to a recipient in the hope that the liver will regenerate and begin to function normally. In fact, the liver does have considerable regenerative capacity, and this may prove a promising approach. The operation, however, is still experimental and rarely performed.

Most cancers in the liver begin somewhere else in the body and spread to the liver. This kind of disease is not curable by a liver transplant. Similarly, tumors that begin in the liver have usually spread to other organs by the time they are detected. This situation will not be changed by liver transplant either. Only diseases that affect the liver alone will be helped by liver transplant. These include, among other diseases and conditions, hepatitis.

Liver transplantation entails all the risks of major surgery and more. The greatest risk is probably not having any liver function for as long as it takes to remove the diseased liver and replace it with a healthy one. After the operation, poor function of the new liver, bleeding, and infection are the major risks.

Some of the immunosuppressant drugs given to prevent rejection of the new organ can lead to infection or the development of tumors. Cortisones produce fluid retention and can worsen diabetes or osteoporosis and promote gastrointestinal bleeding. The immunosuppressant cyclosporine, commonly used in all kinds of transplant operations to prevent rejection, can cause high blood pressure and serious kidney problems. Anyone on immunosuppressants of any kind is more susceptible to infection. And if you have a liver transplant, at least some of these drugs must be taken for the rest of your life.

Careful monitoring is required in the weeks following the operation. Although it varies case by case, most patients will be in the hospital for at least a month after a transplant operation.

Liver transplantation, as you might imagine, is not cheap: including hospitalization, the operation itself, and care over the first year, the average cost is about $300,000, and complicated cases are even more expensive. Continuing care in the ensuing years adds even more to these costs. Medicare does not cover the cost of liver transplants.

Future Treatment

A good deal of research on hepatitis C is currently under way. The National Institutes of Health is studying whether the long-term use of interferon can slow liver damage even in those cases where it doesn't actually eliminate the virus.

There is one new drug being tested, although no results of the test are available as of this writing: Vertex

Pharmaceuticals, a company in Massachusetts, is experimenting with a compound that inhibits the production of a human enzyme called ionosine monophosphate dehydrogenase. The hepatitis C virus apparently relies on this enzyme to make its RNA and reproduce in the human body. If the production of this enzyme can be interfered with in some way, it might be possible to stop the hepatitis C virus from reproducing. In addition, a rather simple treatment is being investigated: taking a pint of blood from hepatitis C patients from time to time. This reduces the amount of iron in the body, and can lower ALT and AST levels. Whether this delays liver damage is still not known.

Some researchers are pursuing a different angle: they are trying to disrupt the process that causes fibrosis. To do this, they are attempting to understand the chemical processes that signal cells to become fibrotic. It is known that the process involves signaling chemicals called cytokines that are released by certain liver cells when they are stimulated by lymphocytes. If this could be interrupted, the destructive effects of hepatitis C might be eliminated or reduced even without eradicating the virus itself.

Of course, the best way to attack hepatitis C would be to find a way to destroy the virus, as we have already done with hepatitis A and B, and, at least to some extent, with HIV. Attacking the protease, helicase, and polymerase enzymes (mentioned in chapter 4) is one way to do this. Another is to develop a drug that will cut the virus's genome. This can be done using short lengths of RNA called ribozymes. But it has proven very difficult to get enough ribozyme to infected cells to accomplish this. A company, aptly named Ribozyme Pharmaceuticals, is working on this approach. Some researchers are using gene therapy techniques to try to make liver cells themselves more resistant to infection by the virus.

6

Living with Hepatitis C

Hepatitis C has infected almost 2 percent of the U.S. population—four million people—and most of them don't even know it. If you are infected, you will very likely have the disease for the rest of your life, since 85 percent of cases of hepatitis C are chronic. This does not mean that you will be incapacitated by it, or even ill. But the infection will very likely remain with you, and you will have to make adjustments in the way you live in order to deal with it.

The worst risk HCV patients face is liver disease. This, of course, can be deadly. But people can be infected with HCV for as long as fifty years without suffering significant liver damage. This does not mean, however, that their quality of life will be the same as someone who does not have HCV.

Sometimes people, including many doctors, minimize the significance of HCV if there is no clinically apparent liver involvement—it is a "benign" infection, it is "indolent," it will be there, but if it doesn't affect your liver you really have little to worry about. Some even ascribe the complaints of HCV patients without liver disease to hypochondria. A British study published in the journal *Hepatology* in January 1998 contradicted this opinion in no uncertain terms. Does an HCV-infected person suffer even if he doesn't have liver disease? The answer is clear, and the answer is yes. In fact, the degree of liver inflammation does not affect the quality of life in HCV infection.

These researchers found that in almost every category—social functioning, physical limitations, mental health, energy and fatigue, pain, and general perception of health—HCV patients were in very bad shape, no matter what their degree of hepatic inflammation. The researchers were careful to eliminate other possible explanations for this: they felt that perhaps drug use, and not HCV, was responsible, but they found that HCV infected people who had not used drugs were scarcely better off than those who had. They guessed that maybe they were seeing only people with other complaints that had nothing to do with HCV, and that that's why the people seemed worse off. But when they compared people who had no complaints but were found by screening to be infected with those who were found to be infected because of a specific complaint, they detected no difference in quality of life. Then they wondered whether the lower quality-of-life scores simply applied to any serious chronic illness, and not to HCV specifically, but when they compared chronic HCV sufferers to chronic HBV patients, the HCV-infected were markedly worse off in every area. And there were no differences in quality of life between those with mild liver inflammation and those with severe liver inflammation, or between those with high ALT levels and those with low levels.

A 1999 American study confirmed this result, demonstrating quite clearly that the degree of impairment of health of people with HCV—even those with no liver disease—was as great as that of people with chronic arthritis or diabetes. This suggests strongly that HCV is not just a liver ailment, but a chronic systemic disease that affects many aspects of health. This study also showed that treatment with interferon improved people's feelings about their health, even when they didn't yet know the results of the blood tests that would show how their liver function was responding. Clearly, treatment provided health benefits not measured by liver function alone.

This means that if you have HCV, even if you don't have liver disease, your quality of life is going to be negatively affected. This chapter presents some ideas about what you can do about it.

Drugs to Avoid or Use with Caution

Many drugs—alcohol, Tylenol, niacin, and high-dose penicillin among others—have an effect on the liver, and people with hepatitis C have to take such drugs very carefully or, if possible, avoid them completely. But it is impossible to simply make a list of drugs that are permitted and drugs that aren't. The picture is much more complicated than that.

Isoniazid, used to treat tuberculosis, can also cause liver damage. Methyldopa, a drug for high blood pressure, can also be poisonous to the liver. The urinary tract infection medicine nitrofurantoin and the antiseizure drug phenytoin can sometimes lead to cirrhosis. In some cases, the statin drugs used to lower cholesterol can also cause liver damage. And there are many other drugs metabolized by the liver that can, in sufficient quantity, cause serious damage, especially to a liver that isn't functioning all that well to begin with.

But this doesn't mean that these drugs are absolutely off limits for all patients. Some tolerate them quite well. Some tolerate them in small doses who could not tolerate them in larger doses. And the benefits of taking the drug must always be weighed in each individual case against the risks of not taking them. For example, aspirin and other anti-inflammatory drugs seem in some cases to lower ALT levels in people with hepatitis. On the other hand, anti-inflammatories reduce the clotting ability of blood, and people with impaired liver function and associated clotting disorders may be harmed by it. Tylenol, suitable in small doses for treating for the flulike symptoms of interferon treatment, may be harmful to the liver in large doses, and people with impaired liver function should probably not take it, since the benefits it offers are not worth the risk. Because Tylenol has these risks, ibuprofen (Motrin or Advil) is sometimes taken by hepatitis C sufferers to combat the joint pain the disease can cause. Physicians may even prescribe it because of Tylenol's bad reputation in liver disease. But this too may be a bad idea. Ibuprofen can also injure the liver—people who take it may see their liver enzymes rise tenfold, which suggests that serious liver damage is occurring. It is even possible that ibuprofen used over time can speed progress toward cirrhosis.

Cigarettes and Nicotine

The many dangers of smoking are well-known and need no discussion here. Nicotine is a poison metabolized by the liver, and a damaged liver metabolizes it more poorly than a healthy one. This can cause nicotine-induced problems throughout the body. Smoking causes circulatory problems, which liver disease victims may already be struggling with. Although some people consider smoking to be less of a problem than alcohol and illicit drugs, it is probably just as important for hepatitis-infected people to avoid nicotine as it is to avoid these other drugs.

Diet

The liver is the most important digestive organ in the body. It metabolizes carbohydrates, fats, and proteins to turn them into substances useful for the body's energy production. It stores vitamins for future use. It filters out material that is harmful, and manufactures enzymes essential to digestion. So when it fails to function properly, the entire body begins to suffer the consequences.

Yet despite what we know about the function of the liver in metabolizing food, much less is known about the effect of diet on liver malfunction, or on a malfunctioning liver. Much is known, for example, and to a high degree of scientific certainty, about the effect of diet on heart disease. There are large prospective studies that offer convincing evidence that a diet low in saturated fat significantly reduces the risk of coronary artery disease and that high serum cholesterol significantly increases it. And many other details about diet and heart disease have been studied. But much less is known for certain about the effect of diet on the liver, perhaps because of this organ's complexity and its multiplicity of functions.

One thing, though, is certain, and at the top of the list for anyone with hepatitis C: you must avoid alcohol. Alcohol speeds the development of liver disease in people infected with hepatitis C. If you drink it, you risk liver damage.

Obesity is a risk in liver disease, because the liver, like other internal organs, gets fat too. In the case of the liver, fat cells can infiltrate it and lead to cirrhosis. It isn't easy to do if you're overweight, but going on a weight-loss diet and exercise program is good for your liver. Only a liver biopsy will tell you if you have fatty infiltra- tion of the liver. Such patients, when they lose weight, almost always see an improvement in their liver enzyme profile. Reducing the percentage of fat in the diet—at least in the early stages of liver disease—is probably also a good idea. High triglyceride levels may lead to in- creased fat deposits in the liver. On the other hand, as liver function deteriorates, high triglycerides and high cholesterol become less of an issue.

People with cirrhosis must avoid high-protein foods, because ammonia levels in the blood will go up on such a diet and may cause coma.

Vitamins

There is growing acceptance in standard medical practice that vitamin supplements have an important role in maintaining health, and many physicians routinely rec- ommend a multivitamin for healthy people. But HCV pa- tients may not benefit from such a regimen, since some vitamins are better than others for these people, and some may even be harmful if taken in sufficient quantity.

Although it doesn't happen commonly, vitamin A can cause liver damage in the doses included in many multivitamins. Symptoms of vitamin A overdose include loss of appetite, headaches, nausea, dry skin, and loss of hair. It may be safer to avoid vitamin A supplements completely in favor of getting the requisite amounts of this vitamin from regular food. Vitamin D in excess, in addition to causing symptoms like those of vitamin A overdose, can also cause depression, constant thirst, and irritability. Excessive intake of iron can cause liver damage, and iron supplements should be avoided by HCV-infected people. It isn't certain, but it may be that excessive iron is a contributor to liver cell mutation.

On the other hand, there are a number of vitamins that can help if you have HCV. B vitamins are good for liver problems. They aid the cytochrome p450 system that controls the way the liver neutralizes harmful material. B1 is often deficient in people afflicted with liver disease, so supplements may be warranted. B6 is also useful—a deficiency of it can impair immune function. Some people feel that injections of B12 are helpful in fighting fatigue.

Vitamin C has probably been oversold as a cure-all, but it is generally harmless, and may be useful in supporting various immune functions. It is also helpful in the formation of collagen, the connective tissue that may be weakened in HCV patients. Calcium is good for improving bone strength.

Glucosamine, which has recently received some publicity as an osteoarthritis treatment, is required for making glycoproteins, essential to digestive processes, and may prove helpful for people with HCV.

Selenium is an important mineral vital to the maintenance of proper immune function, and deficiencies of it can encourage high levels of viral infection. It also aids in the management of fats by the liver, and has some protective effect in alcoholic cirrhosis. The signs of deficiency are somewhat vague—dry skin, dandruff, and fatigue. Cataracts may also be connected to deficiencies of this mineral. Excessive levels can cause problems including fatigue and indigestion.

Vitamin E is an antioxidant useful in combating fatigue, and a deficiency of it may be a cause of poor fat metabolism. Even more significantly, some researchers have concluded that vitamin E helps prevent the molecular changes associated with cirrhosis. Other studies have shown that large doses of vitamin E significantly lower liver enzyme levels when used during interferon therapy. Vitamin K deficiency is also associated with liver disease, and the vitamin is sometimes given by injection to prevent clotting problems associated with deficiency.

You should discuss any of these vitamins with your doctor before you take them, agree on a regimen and dosages, and, as far as possible, carefully monitor their effects in the context of any other treatment you are undergoing.

Food Supplements

Food supplements sold in health food stores vary considerably in quality and price, and few are scientifically proven to be helpful in alleviating the symptoms of HCV or any other liver ailment. (To the extent that they are helpful in alleviating the symptoms of liver disease, however, they could also be used for treating chronic HBV. They are rarely recommended for treating HAV, since that disease goes away by itself, or for treating the nonchronic form of HBV.) Some supplements have been proven to have nutritional qualities, and HCV patients need to pay attention to nutrition perhaps even more carefully than those who are completely healthy. And some HCV patients have surely found these products useful in finding symptomatic relief. Health food store staples such as chlorella (a kind of alga) and kelp (seaweed) have been used by HCV patients. Colloidal silver is said to have antibiotic and antiviral properties. Linseed oil is a source of fatty acids and may have anti-inflammatory properties. Some health food experts recommend extracts from the livers of animals as treatment. Grapefruit seeds, extracts of papaya fruit, shark cartilage, plankton, wheatgrass, and Tibetan yogurt cultures have all been recommended by one practitioner or another. If you use these products, you should read the labels carefully, pay attention to recommended doses, and keep in touch with your doctor about what you are taking and when.

Alternative Medicine: Herbal and Other Remedies for Hepatitis C

There are, of course, other medical traditions than Western scientific medicine. Traditional Chinese medicine depends on the concept of *qi* or *chi*, which has to do with the energy that flows through everything in the universe, including humans and other living organisms. Having this energy flow freely is the key to health, and requires attaining a balance in the body between the well-known yin and yang. Eating certain plants, undergoing acupuncture, and practicing various kinds of exercise are all important in this kind of medicine. Homeopathy is a tradition of treating illnesses with substances that are thought to be similar to the illness itself, such as medications that contain small amounts of the infectious agent that is causing the disease. Naturopathic medicine advocates diet and fasting to promote health, methods thought to be natural processes of healing.

You know if you have read the preceding chapters of this book that Western medicine has only limited solutions to offer people with HCV, so it is to be expected that patients will search elsewhere when conventional treatment fails to provide relief. But note that even the most avid proponent of alternative treatments doesn't recommend any of them for treating hepatitis A. Why not? One reason may be that hepatitis A is well understood scientifically: we know what virus causes it, we can confidently predict the course of the disease, and, most important, we have a highly effective vaccine that prevents it, with almost 100 percent efficacy. To take another example, there are hundreds of "natural" cures for osteoarthritis. This is a common ailment that, scientifically, is poorly understood. There is no scientifically proven cure. And there isn't even any truly effective scientifically proven treatment. Finally—very important—osteoarthritis is a chronic illness that, once they get, people usually suffer with for the rest of their lives. So there is plenty of time, and ample motivation, for people to try just about anything. This is fertile ground for proponents of alternative medicine.

In this respect, hepatitis C is more like osteoarthritis than it is like hepatitis A. Hepatitis C is chronic. Once people get it, they usually have it for a lifetime. There is a treatment, but for many people it isn't very effective. There's no vaccine yet. So there is world enough and time for people to try all sorts of cures that are not proven to cure anything. And of course some of them work—at least in the sense that a person tries something, feels better, and then attributes the improvement to whatever it is he tried. With enough publicity—a radio interview here, a TV show there, and a book that's placed in the window of Barnes & Noble—this treatment, however scientifically dubious, becomes the latest alternative medicine for hepatitis C.

This is not to say that there are no herbal remedies or alternative treatments that might have a positive effect on hepatitis C. Milk thistle, for example, a plant extract taken orally, is recommended by some for the illness, and has actually been shown in some cases to reduce certain liver enzyme levels in infected people. And of course many vegetables have positive effects on health. But there are few scientific studies of the effectiveness of milk thistle extract in combating hepatitis C; there are no clinical trials to suggest which patients it might work for; there are no regulations concerning its purity or concentration, which may vary considerably from one batch to another; no one knows the proper dosage quantities; and there is little knowledge of its side effects, drug interactions, or other possible dangers.

Herbs are in any case difficult to study. They have so many chemicals in them that it's very hard to know which is causing a desired effect, which is causing a harmful effect, and which is causing no effect at all. Assertions about the effectiveness of herbs for medical treatment often rely on anecdotal evidence, some of it, to be sure, gathered over many years or even centuries, but still only anecdotal. On the other hand, anecdotal reports of the effectiveness of a given remedy are often what inspire researchers to test a substance for effectiveness using standard scientific methods.

The FDA does not review the safety and effectiveness of herbal medicines, nor does it regulate their labeling or advertising. There is a law, the Dietary Supplement Health and Education Act of 1994, that makes it illegal to market herbal products for the diagnosis, treatment, cure, or prevention of any disease. This explains, at least in part, why the manufacturers' assertions for their herbal preparations are sometimes so vague that they seem to be "good for whatever ails you."

Although there is no American regulation of herbal medicine, there is a German government agency that conducts assessments of the peer-reviewed literature on herbal remedies. This agency, commonly referred to as Commission E, has issued reports on about three hundred herbal medicines, and these reports are considered among the best information available. In addition to these, Phytopharm U.S. Institute of Phytopharmaceuticals has reviewed literature on an additional three hundred remedies. All of these herbs are listed in a very useful reference, *The Physicians' Desk Reference for Herbal Medicines*, and we rely here on those listings. There are five different herbal remedies recommended specifically for the treatment of hepatitis. A description of each follows.

Milk thistle. This is the plant most often recommended by herbalists for the treatment of liver ailments. It is indigenous to Europe, and the ripe seeds of the plant contain the medicinal properties. The plant contains various compounds, but the one that apparently has the effect on liver disease is silymarin, which acts as an antidote to various liver toxins. Silymarin acts on liver cells to make them impenetrable to certain poisons, and stimulates the production of new liver cells. In addition to being used to treat chronic liver inflammation and cirrhosis, silymarin is an antidote to death-cap mushroom poisoning.

Milk thistle (sometimes called Marian thistle) is usually prepared by dissolving 3 grams of the drug in water, boiling it for ten to twenty minutes, and then drinking the infusion. The daily dose is 12 to 15 grams of the drug, or the equivalent of about 300 mg of silymarin. There are no known health risks in using the plant.

Rue. Like many herbal remedies, rue is said to be effective for many different ailments, among them hepatitis. But its primary use is for menstrual disorders and as an abortive agent. The plant is also recommended for inflammations of the skin and mouth tissue, earache, toothache, and stomach problems. The plant contains dozens of chemicals, which may help to explain its varied actions. It can be dangerous for pregnant women, or if taken in incorrect dosages. It is ingested as a tea or applied topically to the skin or other affected area, including as an eardrop and as a filling for toothaches. The entire plant is used medicinally, including its flowers and oils extracted from the herb. When taken internally, the dose is 0.5 to 1 gram daily.

Blackcurrant. This too is a plant said to be effective for many problems: arthritis, gout, rheumatism, bladder stones, diarrhea, whooping cough, inflammations of the mouth and throat, urinary problems, wounds, insect bites—and hepatitis. The dried-out leaves and the fresh ripe fruit (often freeze-dried for distribution) contain the medicinal properties. The plant is indigenous to Europe, Asia, Canada, and Australia, and is cultivated elsewhere. Holland, Poland, France, Hungary, and the former Yugoslavia are the chief exporters of the product. The medicine is administered as a tea internally and as a compress externally. Three to four cups of the tea are drunk per day, each containing about 3 grams of blackcurrant leaves. No side effects are known to occur when the plant is used in the recommended dosages, but people with edema resulting from reduced heart or kidney function should not use it.

Licorice. This is another plant that is used for many ailments—the roots and runners of the plant are used as medicine for coughs and bronchitis, upper respiratory tract infections, and gastric or duodenal ulcers. One of its chemical ingredients, glycyrrhizic acid, is used in the treatment of viral liver inflammation, but it is contraindicated in cases of chronic hepatitis and cirrhosis. It apparently works by inducing the production of interferon. No side effects are known when it is used in other instances.

Soybean. The main action of soybean is in reducing levels of cholesterol, but it is also used in nutritional liver diseases and in chronic hepatitis. It is taken in an oral preparation that consists of an average daily dose of 1.5 to 3.5 grams of phospholipids from soybeans. Stomach pain, loose stool, and diarrhea are among the side effects, but no other health hazards are known when the product is used in the recommended dosages.

In addition to these "officially approved" plants, there are studies of other herbal remedies that seem to show some effectiveness in the treatment of liver disease. In one such study a Chinese research team looked at the effects of bing gan ling oral liquid for treating hepatitis C. Bing gan ling is a liquid made of various plants and roots (*Cornu bubali, Rhizoma polygoni cuspidati, Radix paeoniae Rubra*) that is said to "cool" the blood and regulate the functioning of the liver and spleen. A study of sixty patients with chronic hepatitis C infection showed that the preparation did actually have some effectiveness in lowering liver enzyme levels.

Dozens of plants, usually ones that are not normally used in Western cuisines, are recommended by herbalists as treatments for hepatitis C. Some may have beneficial effects such as reducing inflammation, increasing appetite, and decreasing fluid retention that could be helpful for people suffering from HCV and from many other diseases as well. Indeed, as we have seen, the same plants that are recommended for treating hepatitis C are also used by herbalists and other practitioners for treating dozens of other ailments.

Many of the plants recommended are said to "detoxify" or "enhance" the immune system, claims whose vagueness makes them very difficult to refute. Among others that are said to do this are aloe vera, burdock root, barberry, kombucha (a Chinese mushroom), garlic, sileris (a Chinese herb), pau d'arco (a South American herb), *Astragalus membranaceus* (huang chi), and *Fungus japonicus* (a Japanese mushroom).

Similarly vague are the claims that certain plants "detoxify the liver" or "purify the blood," contentions that are almost impossible to systematically reject because the meaning of these phrases is so nonspecific. Among these are burdock root, garden celandine, *Desmodium ascendens* (an African herb), isatis root (ban lan gen, a Chinese plant), peony root, yellow dock, sarsaparilla, and dandelion roots and leaves.

Some plants are recommended for problems of blood circulation: ginkgo biloba (maidenhair tree), *Radix angelicae* (angelica root, pang gui, dong quai), and white peony root. Others are said to reduce fluid retention: black snakeroot (*Cimifuga racemosa*), artichokes (leaves, stems, and roots), *Rhizoma atartylodis* (bai zhu, pai shu, a Chinese herb), the roots of *A. membranaceus* (huang chi), and St. John's wort (which has recently attained some notoriety in the treatment of depression) are all said to do this.

Anti-inflammatory properties are said to be shown by wild yam, purple coneflower, and isatis root (ban lan gen).

Some plants have been shown to lower liver enzymes in animal testing: the mushrooms *Grifola frondosa, Lentinus erodus*, and *Tricholoma lobayense*, for example. It should be noted that mushrooms (and this goes for *F. japonicus* mentioned above as well) can be very dangerous even to healthy people, and that if you use these, you should be extremely cautious about which mushrooms you ingest.

Many plants are recommended as general all-around treatments for hepatitis or liver malfunction: garden celandine, *Echinops grijisii* and *Eclipta prostata* (Taiwanese folk remedies), *Eleutherococcus senticosus* (Siberian ginseng), Oregon grape root, *Swertia mileensis* (a Chinese folk medicine), *Cnicus benedictus* (holy thistle or blessed thistle), Chinese bupleurum, California buckthorn, and peony root.

Herbalists rarely claim that plants actually destroy the virus, but there are some exceptions: barberry, coptis root (huang lian, a Chinese herb), St. John's wort, and chaparral are all said to have antiviral properties.

If you are going to use herbal remedies, it is important to inform your doctor of which ones you're trying. If liver function deteriorates while you are using them, you will want to stop them for a time to see if they are causing the problem. There are certain herbs recommended by some for hepatitis C that should definitely be avoided. These include sho-saiko-to, a traditional Japanese remedy; Jin Bu Huan Anodyne, a Chinese herbal preparation; glycyrrhizin, a Chinese herbal tea; oil of cloves; comfrey tea; T'suanchi'I, a Chinese tonic; and Asian ginseng (*Panax ginseng*). All of these have been implicated in causing liver disease.

You will of course use natural remedies if you are inclined to do so. They may do some good, and most, if not used excessively or to the exclusion of other nutrients, can do no harm. But use them carefully. Tell your doctor what you are taking. Keep abreast of new developments—many of these treatments are being tested more systematically, and the results of this research may be useful. And remember: just because a treatment is "natural" does not mean it is necessarily safe or effective.

7

Hepatitis D
THE DELTA VIRUS

In 1977 a researcher working in Turin, Italy, with the blood of HBV-infected patients found what was first thought to be a new HBV antigen. But on further study, it was determined that what the researcher had found was a new virus entirely, yet another form of hepatitis virus, and the oddest one yet. This one, named the delta virus, and now usually called hepatitis D, cannot exist without the hepatitis B virus. The two infections can be contracted at once—called coinfection—or a hepatitis B sufferer can get hepatitis D infection in addition—superinfection. Since you can't get HDV unless you get HBV, there is a nearly 100 percent effective preventive step you can take: get vaccinated for HBV. But if you already have HBV, you are susceptible to HDV, and there is so far no vaccine against it, nor a truly effective treatment for it.

The interactions between HBV and HDV are poorly understood, but the two probably act together to make the disease worse and liver disease more serious. HDV

Geographic distribution of HDV infection

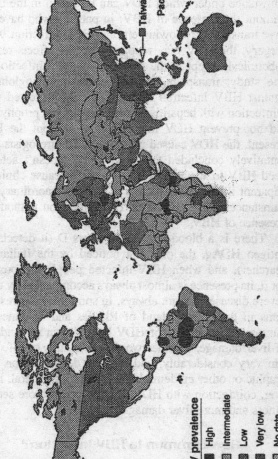

HDV prevalence
- High
- Intermediate
- Low
- Very low
- No data

Pacific islands

Taiwan

usually, but not always, causes liver damage. In fact, in people infected with both HBV and HDV, it is the HDV that is probably doing the most harm. There is one circumstance under which HDV can be found in the blood without the presence of HBV: in patients who have had liver transplants following chronic HBV infection. After surgery, the HDV may reappear, but its effects remain subclinical except in the presence of HBV infection. In one study, transplant patients given immunoglobulins against HBV infection were effectively protected from reinfection with hepatitis B, even though the prophylaxis did not prevent HDV infection. But without the HBV present, the HDV caused no disease. So virologists have tentatively concluded that while HDV doesn't actually need HBV to survive, it does need it to cause clinically apparent illness. Still, except in these extraordinary circumstances, there can be no HDV infection without the presence of HBV.

There is a blood test for hepatitis D (it detects the antigen HDAg, the one first noticed by the Italian researcher), and when HBV-infected people are positive for it, its presence is almost always accompanied by more severe disease. But not always. In some recent investigations in the Greek island of Rhodes and in American Samoa, many carriers of HDV have shown no evidence of liver damage. In other words, the results of infection can vary considerably, and may be dependent on geographic or other epidemiologic factors. In general, however, coinfection with HDV usually means more serious illness and more liver damage.

How Common Is HDV Infection?

A rough estimate is that about 6 percent of the total chronic disease burden due to hepatitis can be attributed to HDV. The prevalence of the disease in the general population (this can be estimated by checking blood donors for the virus) is between about 1.4 and 8 percent, but people who have had repeated through-the-skin exposures have much higher rates. Injection drug users have rates that vary from 20 to 53 percent, depending on the population studied, and hemophilia patients have even higher rates: 48 to 80 percent. In populations where the high rate of HBV infection is due to transmission during infancy or childhood (Alaskan Natives and Eskimos, for example), HDV is practically nonexistent.

HDV is endemic in the Mediterranean basin (particularly in Italy), the Middle East, South America, West Africa, and some South Pacific islands. In these areas of high endemicity, HDV infection accounts for a significant proportion of liver transplants.

The prevalence of HDV tends to be lower in areas with temperate and cold climates than in tropical and subtropical countries. Although a higher rate of HBV infection usually means higher HDV rates, it doesn't always. In fact, in many countries where HBV is common, HDV nevertheless remains rare. Still, where you control the rates of HBV, HDV also declines, as has happened in Europe in recent years. Measures to control HIV have also had the side benefit of controlling rates of HBV and HDV.

What Happens to People with HDV Infection

Clinically, a person infected with HDV at first doesn't look any different from other hepatitis patients—only a blood test will reveal the infection. But the disease then takes its toll. In about 15 percent of patients the illness progresses to liver failure quite quickly—within a few months to a year or two. But in most people it is asymptomatic for many years. Typically, injection drug users are among that 15 percent; people who live in endemic areas are in the majority whose disease progresses more slowly. Still, within a few years, these patients begin to develop cirrhosis. At this point, when cirrhosis is evident, HDV replication decreases to a point where the blood test isn't sensitive enough to detect it, and the patient can remain stable for a period of many years.

While HBV can sometimes infect tissues other than the liver—the pancreas or peripheral blood cells, for example—HDV has never been demonstrated to infect any cells other than liver cells.

Cirrhosis develops quite quickly in many HDV patients. An Italian study showed that 40 percent of HDV-infected adults and 30 percent of HDV-infected children had progressed to cirrhosis within two to six years. The kind of damage HDV does to the liver is indistinguishable on biopsy from the damage done by other forms of hepatitis infection. Other studies suggest, however, that even though this is so, chronic HBV-HDV infection leads to no more liver failure or liver cancer than chronic HBV infection alone. Still, 70 percent of HDV-infected people develop some sort of cirrhosis, and the disease can be deadly: mortality rates range from 2 to 20 percent, depending on the population studied.

Treatment

Treatment by means other than liver transplant is discouraging. The only drug currently used for HDV, recombinant interferon, does not work well for most patients. Experiments have shown that in cultures of HDV without the presence of HBV, HDV is resistant to interferon, so any benefit attained by HDV-infected patients using interferon probably comes from reducing the number of host HBV viruses present in the blood. Using interferon is the only choice for the moment, but its use is frustrating: if it is used, it must be given over substantial periods of time to have any chance of success, but there are no real reference points to aid in deciding whether the drug has worked or whether therapy should be discontinued at a given time. When HDV is treated with interferon, there is usually some inhibition of replication, but relapses are common, and inflammation of the liver is not often diminished—another suggestion that the interferon may be working against HBV while leaving HDV to do the liver damage. When interferon is stopped, most patients relapse within a few months.

Lamivudine, a nucleoside analogue that has some effect in treating HBV, has been tested for treating HDV as well. In one study, patients were given 100 mg of the drug orally once a day for a year. Serum levels of HBV DNA fell, but the patients remained HBsAg and HDV RNA positive. The drug had no effect on the progression of disease, so it has turned out to be not very useful.

It is difficult at present to make any recommendations about the best way to treat HDV infection. Interferon has not been approved for this purpose, but many doctors and their patients will want to try it anyway. The dose should be started at 5 μ daily or 9–10 μ three times a week, and this level should be decreased only if it is not tolerated. Regular blood tests every two to four weeks should be done during the therapy for blood count and aminotransferase. Every three to four months, thyroid and liver function, bilirubin, albumin, and total protein should be examined. If there is no improvement in ALT levels after three months, interferon should not be continued, but if there is improvement, the therapy should go on for at least a year. At this point, if HBsAg is negative, there will probably be a sustained response to the treatment.

There have been some attempts to produce a vaccine against HDV, with some promising results but no definitive success, in animal studies. There is no vaccine that has been tested in humans. Virologists now believe that they can plan a pharmacological attack against the virus by designing a drug that will interfere with its RNA replication, but so far no drug has been effective in doing this.

If there is any good news in this picture, it is that liver transplants work well—the new liver is less often reinfected after the operation than it is with other forms of hepatitis. In fact, for some reason, patients who are infected with both HDV and HBV do better after transplant than those infected with HBV alone. In these patients HDV appears to survive for a time when HBV is suppressed with anti-HBs immunoglobulin after transplantation, and then the HDV gradually disappears. Underlying HDV infection doesn't usually cause problems unless and until HBV superinfection returns. Five-year survival rates for HDV patients with transplanted livers can range as high as 88 percent.

The only truly effective attack now against HDV is prevention, and the best tool by far for prevention of HDV is the vaccine for HBV. In Italy, rates have been reduced substantially by a program of universal vaccination with the HBV vaccine. The people who are currently infected were infected years ago, and survived the immediate medical effects of HDV. While the disease has remained asymptomatic in some, in the majority it has advanced to cirrhosis but then subsided after that. The number of new cases is vastly reduced. Obviously, reductions in intravenous drug use and careful screening of the blood supply are also required. Vaccinating high-risk groups has not, however, proven to be an effective strategy, and the CDC now recommends that hepatitis B vaccine be included in routine childhood vaccination programs.

Transmission

Although HDV is a virus passed among people with HBV, beyond that the modes of transmission are not clear. It is certainly true that it is transmitted in blood and blood products, both by transfusion and by infected injection equipment. But there is also some evidence that it can be transmitted within families. In a study done in Italy, the molecular structure of HDV RNA gathered from family members—mothers, sisters, and brothers—clearly indicated that they were infected with the same strain of the virus. This almost certainly means that the virus can be transmitted through personal contact, and not just by transfusion or needle sharing. Of course, the family member must be infected with HBV before being infected with HDV. The study did not suggest how the transmission might have taken place, but only that some sort of personal contact is quite clearly a route of transmission.

HDV can be transmitted sexually, though its transmission by this route is less efficient than that of HBV. It can be transmitted either as a coinfection along with HBV or as a superinfection to someone already infected with HBV. In homosexual men, transmission rates increase with the number of partners and with the frequency of anal intercourse. Among female prostitutes, the rate of HDV infection in a recent study was 15 percent, somewhat higher for those who used injection drugs, somewhat lower for those who did not. Sexual transmission also occurs from drug users to their sexual partners.

In the United States as a whole, there are approximately 70,000 carriers of HDV, and the virus kills approximately 1,000 people per year.

A Virus Unlike Any Other

HDV is a class of animal viruses new to biologists. In some ways it more closely resembles viruses that infect plants than those that infect animals. Chimpanzees can be infected with it, and woodchucks have also been used in experimenting with the virus. It infects humans with a vengeance—about ten million people worldwide, all of them infected with HBV as well, have the delta virus.

Viruses need an envelope around them in order to survive, and the hepatitis D virus depends on the hepatitis B virus to supply its envelope. In fact, the envelope of hepatitis D is actually made of hepatitis B surface antigen (HBsAg). Once wrapped in this envelope, HDV manufactures a protein, hepatitis D antigen (HDAg) and viral RNA, which it uses to replicate. Other than using this bit of hepatitis B surface antigen, its function is independent of HBV.

There are three different genotypes of HDV (slight variations in the genetic structure of the virus particle), and they have different geographic distributions. Genotype I is most common in North America and Italy; genotype II in Japan and Taiwan; and genotype III exists only in northern South America. The significance of the three genotypes to severity of disease is not clear, except that there is apparently an association between genotype III and more severe forms of fulminant infection.

But it gets even stranger: HDV seems to reduce the serological markers of HBV—even though the disease gets worse with HDV coinfection. HBsAg and HBV DNA are both reduced in patients who are coinfected with HDV. So while HBV helps HDV replicate, at the same time HDV seems to inhibit the replication of HBV. Understanding these mechanisms may well be important to developing drugs and other therapies for chronic HBV. So far, biologists know little about them.

Under experimental conditions it is possible to infect a cell line from chimpanzees or woodchucks with HDV without the presence of HBV, but this involves bypassing the processes of cell penetration that the presence of HBV allows HDV to perform in infected people. This can only be done in a laboratory, but of course it is useful for studying the virus. It is one way, for example, that the effect of a given drug on HDV can be tested. In fact, most of our knowledge of the molecular biology of HDV has come from using this laboratory procedure, known as "transfection" to distinguish it from the natural process of infection.

HDV looks a little like some plant viruses in its structure and in the way it reproduces, but it is different enough from any other virus that biologists have had to invent a new classification for it: *Deltaviridae*, a genus of which HDV is the only member.

Geography and the Severity of HDV Disease

It is known that HDV infection makes HBV infection more severe and causes more liver damage. But the degree of increased severity varies depending on where in the world you are. In South America, for example, there have been particularly bad outbreaks of HDV because the genotype dominant there causes more serious disease. But despite many animal experiments designed to figure this out, exactly what characteristic of the virus makes it more severe in some cases and less in others is still not known.

There is some suggestion that the immune response of the infected person may be a factor in how severe HDV infection is, and some signs of autoimmune activity have been detected in the blood of HDV-infected people. But there is no proof, and the significance of immune responses to the virus is still unknown.

Many Questions

As you may have already gathered, much remains unknown about the delta virus. Is the damage caused by HDV due to an immune response, or does the virus itself poison and destroy the cells of the liver? Do the different strains of the virus completely account for its variable effects in different people and in different parts of the world? What is the nature of the relationship between the delta virus and the hepatitis B virus? Why does D require the presence of B to cause clinical illness? Is there a way to vaccinate carriers of hepatitis B against hepatitis D? Why doesn't interferon work to prevent HDV replication? All of these questions, and more, remain to be answered.

8

Hepatitis E

In 1955, in New Delhi, India, 29,000 people became ill with an unknown virus that was apparently infecting the city's water supply. No one knew what it was until the early 1980s, at which time researchers began to study this and other epidemics of waterborne hepatitis cases in India, using the then newly developed antibody tests for hepatitis A, and assuming that that would be the virus they would find. But they found no antibodies for hepatitis A, leading them to conclude, quite correctly, that they had discovered a new form of viral hepatitis. They called it hepatitis E. By 1983 they had made a molecular identification of this new organism, and transmitted the virus experimentally to nonhuman primates. The monkeys were inoculated with feces from patients in an outbreak of hepatitis E in Tashkent. The monkeys got sick, and the viral particles recovered from the sick monkeys were similar to the particles in the human victims of the disease. This made the identification solid: the virus was clearly associated with disease because it was present only in infected sources, and it clearly elicited an antibody response in infected people. Eventually, scientists were able to actually see the virus using electron microscopy.

Hepatitis E infects not just people, but various species of monkeys, rodents, pigs, and chickens as well. This may help to explain why the disease is endemic in certain parts of the world: people and animals, in places where sanitation is substandard, share the same water supplies, and probably pass the virus back and forth between them.

There are at least two strains of HEV, called the HEV-Burma and HEV-Mexico, and there are some subgroups of these strains as well, with slightly different genetic makeup.

The Epidemics and the Disease

On the molecular level, little is known about the precise mechanisms by which HEV infects people, because it's very hard to culture HEV and propagate it in a laboratory. But on the epidemiological level a good deal is known. HEV infects a large number of people in endemic areas, and is especially deadly among pregnant women. Fecal contamination of drinking water is usually the cause, and epidemics have been reported in Nepal, Pakistan, Burma, parts of the former Soviet Union, India, Borneo, Somalia, Sudan, and China. There has been only one documented outbreak in North America—in Mexico in 1986, when some two hundred cases were reported in two neighboring towns to the south of Mexico City.

In western Europe and in North America, confirmed cases of HEV have been traced to immigrants or tourists from endemic countries. Travelers even to endemic regions do not often contract the illness, but where symp-

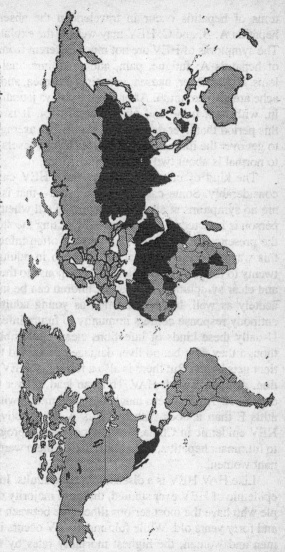

Geographic distribution of hepatitis E

Outbreaks or confirmed infection in more than 25% of sporadic non-ABC hepatitis

toms of hepatitis occur in travelers in the absence of hepatitis A, B, and C, HEV may well be the explanation. The symptoms of HEV are not much different from those of hepatitis A: fatigue, pain, and gastrointestinal problems. Chills, fever, nausea, vomiting, diarrhea, and headache are also common. After about ten days jaundice sets in, with dark urine and clay-colored stool. It is during this period that liver damage can occur. The average time to get over the illness and have liver enzyme levels return to normal is about two months.

The kind of infection you get from HEV can vary considerably. Some cases are subclinical—that is, there are no symptoms at all. The only way to tell whether the person is infected in such cases is by testing the stool for the presence of the virus. Children are often infected in this way. In acute cases, more common in adults aged twenty to forty, there is an antibody response to the virus, and clear symptoms of disease. Children can be infected acutely as well, but not as often as young adults. The antibody response confers immunity to future infections. Usually these kinds of infections clear, and, unpleasant though they may be, no liver damage occurs and the patient gets better. But there is also a fulminant HEV infection, as there is with HAV. This can lead to liver failure and death. This happens much more commonly with hepatitis E than it does with hepatitis A. In a study of an HEV epidemic in China, 9 percent of people progressed to fulminant hepatitis, and almost half of them were pregnant women.

Like HAV, HEV is a disease of young adults. In every epidemic of HEV ever studied, the large majority of people who have the most serious illness are between twenty and forty years old. While fulminant HEV occurs in both men and women, the highest mortality rates by far are among women in their third trimester of pregnancy. The mortality rate for pregnant women in the third trimester is near 20 percent, a finding that is consistent in all epidemics regardless of geography.

For reasons no one understands, the longer a woman has been pregnant, the more likely she is to die from acute hepatitis E. While poor nutrition among pregnant women in developing countries has been suggested as a cause for this, there is no proof that this is so.

The Transmission of HEV

HEV is spread by oral contact with infected fecal matter. It doesn't occur by transmission from person to person, and it probably isn't carried by contact with blood or blood products. There is a possibility that transfused blood could carry the virus in certain stages of infection, but studies of hemophiliacs who receive regular blood transfusions demonstrate that this must be extremely rare. While we know that pregnant women are more susceptible than others to infection, we don't know much about how, or even whether, the virus is transmitted from mothers to their newborns. This is an area in which much more research is required.

A Vaccine for HEV?

Because macaque monkeys experience and recover from HEV infection in very much the same way as humans, scientists have a good animal model to work with. And in fact, a vaccine that appears to work for monkeys has been developed. It is conceivable that the vaccine can be developed for use in endemic areas and for travelers to those areas in the near future, but so far no vaccine is available.

Protecting Yourself from HEV

Since there is no vaccine for HEV, avoidance of the virus is the only way to prevent the disease. Person-to-person transmission does not appear to occur, unlike with hepatitis A. Pregnant women and their unborn babies run the greatest risk for mortality, but not much is known about the transmission of fulminant HEV from mothers to their children. Small studies have suggested that it does occur, and that it can be deadly for the child.

In endemic areas, the best defense against HEV is a clean water supply. If you don't travel to endemic areas, you are extremely unlikely to contract hepatitis E, and you are only slightly more likely to contract it if you do. No case of hepatitis E in North America or western Europe has ever been traced to anything except immigrants and tourists from endemic areas—the virus is otherwise nonexistent in these regions. In fact, there have been only four documented cases of HEV in people in the United States, all of whom had recently traveled to or lived in endemic areas. It is important to remember that there are two groups most at risk for the dangerous fulminant form of the illness: pregnant women, and people between the ages of fifteen and forty.

9

Hepatitis G and Beyond

Unfortunately, the hepatitis story does not end with the depredations now being caused by hepatitis C and chronic hepatitis B. Virologists are finding that there are still more viruses that attack the liver, viruses that so far have not presented a serious health threat, but may in the future.

Hepatitis G

Hepatitis G is one of these. It is similar to the hepatitis C virus, another member of the flavivirus family. The virus can be detected by using the polymerase chain reaction test to detect viral RNA in infected fluids or tissue.

The existence of the virus was confirmed in 1995 when it was cloned from the plasma of a patient who was infected with HCV. A second clone was obtained from a phlebotomist who had apparently contracted the virus in the course of his work and who had no other hepatitis viruses in his blood.

HGV infection tends to exist along with other kinds of hepatitis infection. In fact, there are rarely cases of hepatitis G infection with no other kind of hepatitis present. The Centers for Disease Control has found that about 10 to 15 percent of people with HCV also have HGV RNA in their blood. The prevalence of the disease in the general population is still unknown, but preliminary estimates are that as many as 1.6 percent of volunteer blood donors have HGV RNA in their blood. HGV is spread in the same way as other bloodborne viruses—there have been documented cases of transmission by blood transfusion, for example. There is at least one report of the virus possibly being spread by sexual contact, but no proof at all that this is a common or even possible means of transmission.

A recent study looked at a small number of patients who had liver disease but no A, B, or C hepatitis infection. In three of five cases of acute hepatitis, hepatitis G was present, as it was in three of twenty-three cases of chronic liver disease and in one of seven cases of hepatocellular carcinoma. These results are hardly overwhelming, and certainly not definitive evidence of a clinical effect of hepatitis G, but they may suggest that the virus can, under certain circumstances, be a cause of liver disease. There may be other explanations for hepatitis in people without infections of A, B, or C, and virologists are trying to track them down.

An Explanation for Non-A, Non-E Hepatitis?

An Italian researcher named Daniele Primi works in a research lab run by a company called Diasorin in Brescia. Although the company has not submitted his work to a peer-reviewed journal, it has applied for patents for the discovery of a new hepatitis virus, called S.E.N.-V after the initials of the person in whose blood it was first found (the V stands for "virus"), and for the tests to identify it. Using stored blood samples from patients with hepatitis that does not appear to be caused by hepatitis A through E, the National Institutes of Health is now looking for the new virus as well. If Primi's results can be confirmed—and most scientists believe they can be—then the question of screening blood and blood products for the new virus will become urgent. This new virus may explain those cases of hepatitis that are now called "non A, non E"—cases, that is, that presently available tests all come up negative for, even though hepatitis is clinically present.

Identifying this new virus is the first step. Then researchers will have to determine how many cases of hepatitis are caused by it, whether it can be spread by sexual or other contact as well as by the transfusion of blood products, what effect the virus has on other forms of hepatitis infection and on AIDS, and what role the virus plays in other diseases such as fulminant forms of hepatitis A and B. Researchers will also want to know if some healthy people carry the virus without showing symptoms of disease.

Primi's method was to take samples of HIV-infected, and therefore immunosuppressed, blood, in which he suspected that other viruses might find a home. By testing hundreds of such samples, he was able to discover something he believed was a hepatitis-causing virus. Then he looked again for the virus in samples of blood from non-A, non-E patients. Given a group of coded samples of non-A, non-E infected people and of healthy people as controls, he tested them all, without knowing which were which. The virus turned up in a large percentage of the non-A, non-E sample, but in few of the healthy ones.

The case has not been proven yet. Other viruses have been thought to cause non-A, non-E hepatitis, but then further research eliminated them as possible agents. This could still happen with S.E.N.-V. On the other hand, Dr. Primi may be onto something.

10

Future Medicine
RESEARCH ON HEPATITIS

Large amounts of government and private research money are being poured into virology research. In July 1999, for example, the National Institute of Diabetes and Digestive and Kidney Diseases, a part of the National Institutes of Health, funded a $28 million, eight-year-long clinical trial to research the long-term drug treatment of hepatitis C patients. The study will begin in 2000 at nine different trial centers across the country in an attempt to see if drug treatment can slow the progression of liver disease in these patients. The studies will be undertaken at the University of California at Irvine, the University of Southern California, the University of Colorado Health Sciences Center, Massachusetts General Hospital, the University of Massachusetts Medical School, St. Louis University, the University of Michigan, the University of Texas Southwestern Medical Center, and the Medical College of Virginia.

One of the problems in doing research on hepatitis C is that until recently it has been impossible to culture the virus. But in 1999 German researchers managed to engineer the genes of the hepatitis C virus so that it will replicate in human cells used for research. If this cell line can be reproduced in other labs, it will allow researchers to follow the life cycle of the virus in greater detail, and to try drugs against it until they find one that has an antiviral effect. If this effect is found, they can then test the drug in animals and finally in patients. Needless to say, an essential step in this process will be for a pharmaceutical company to buy up the licenses for the drugs that work and patent any patentable processes by which they are used or manufactured.

Protease inhibitors, drugs that interfere with the production of proteins necessary to viral reproduction (see chapter 4 for a discussion of the life cycle of the hepatitis C virus), are another promising possibility. These drugs are already used with some success in combating HIV, and they may find a role in defeating HCV and chronic HBV as well. Making the protease inhibitors effective requires a detailed knowledge of the structure of the virus, because these drugs work by attaching themselves to specific sites on the virus, like a wrench that fits perfectly around a bolt. Unfortunately, protease inhibitors, in disrupting the reproduction of viruses, often disrupt the workings of normal cells as well, causing unpleasant side effects. In fact, the HIV protease inhibitors cause their worst side effects in patients with liver disease, a rather discouraging fact when considering their use in fighting HCV.

It has recently been discovered that the reason interferon works only poorly with genotype 1 of HCV is that this genotype contains a protein called E2, lacking in other types, that inactivates an enzyme that is essential to interferon's effectiveness. Interferon works by making one of the body's enzymes, PKR, block the virus's ability to attach itself to a cell. E2 from the virus counters this defense. Knowledge of this mechanism, combined with the ability to culture HCV in the laboratory, may lead to better drugs in the future.

One new area of drug research concerns ribozymes. Ribozymes are proteins that function as a kind of molecular scissors—they are capable of cutting RNA in a gene, effectively turning the gene off so that its effect can be studied. (Their discoverer, Thomas Cech, won the Nobel Prize for Chemistry in 1989.) Ribozymes had been considered mostly as a research tool in genetics, but therapeutic applications are now being developed—for instance, in cutting the RNA of genes that produce disease, making them inoperable. There is also some indication that perhaps ribozymes could be used to cut viral RNA, making it ineffective. One company has developed a ribozyme called Heptazyme that targets the RNA of the HCV virus. This drug is still under development and not yet at the stage of clinical trials.

Directions for Future Research

There is much to be learned about the epidemiology of hepatitis, particularly of hepatitis C. Many things are still unclear: why the disease is more prevalent among poor people, what the modes of transmission are within households, what are the mechanisms of sexual transmission, or the specifics of perinatal transmission. Long-term studies are needed to try to determine what factors in hepatitis lead to cirrhosis, why some people progress quickly to liver damage and others don't. Why do some patients appear to have normal levels of ALT even though they are infected with hepatitis C? What is the prognosis for the treatment of people coinfected with HIV and HCV? No one understands completely the role of ultrasound or alpha-fetoprotein levels in detecting early hepatocellular cancer in people with hepatitis C.

Why do some people clear hepatitis from their systems after treatment with interferon and ribavirin, while others continue to be infected? No one knows. Everyone knows that drinking alcohol helps hepatitis destroy the liver, but no one knows exactly what the mechanism is. Nor do we understand completely the relationship of obesity, diabetes, iron, and various medications to the progress of cirrhosis.

As you know if you read chapter 4, the interpretation of the tests that indicate hepatitis C infection are prone to a great deal of subjectivity if not outright guessing. How can these tests be used to decide what kind of treatment is best? Which is the best test? What is the significance of variations in results in the same person at different times? What about people who test positive on the RIBA test but negative for HCV RNA?

Little is known about the disease in people under eighteen or over sixty, and clinical trials for these groups, as well as minority populations, are essential. Large clinical trials may also help to clarify the best procedure for people who do not respond to interferon therapy or who relapse after therapy is concluded. Also needed are prospective studies to identify the factors that predict response to therapy. Drug interactions are another area that requires extensive examination, especially in figuring out the interactions between drugs used to treat hepatitis and the antivirals used to treat HIV.

Prevention efforts remain vitally important. Education among risk groups and screening of blood, organs, tissue, and semen must continue. The best way to prevent disease, of course, is vaccination, and the search for a safe and effective vaccine against hepatitis C is the most important scientific quest in this area.

New Drugs

Getting a new drug to market is difficult, even after the complex work of discovering which drug has promise against a given illness. Drug companies, the National Institutes of Health, and large universities all fund this research, testing new drugs that are then submitted to the Food and Drug Administration for approval. This is a long and demanding process.

After researchers have found an antiviral drug, they test it on animals. This step assures the safety and predicts the effectiveness of the drug, as well as establishing the parameters for dosage in humans. After this testing meets with success—that is, after the drug demonstrates some success in treating the disease in lab animals—the FDA must approve the drug for clinical trials in humans. This is a three-step process.

In Phase I, the drug is tested for toxicity. With a small number of volunteers (usually both people who are ill and healthy controls), the drug is given in varying amounts, and its effects are carefully monitored—its rate of absorption, how it moves through the body, and how it is metabolized and eliminated. In Phase II, larger numbers of patients are studied to see how the drug works in varying dosages over time and to gather preliminary evidence of efficacy. Phase III tests hundreds, sometimes thousands, of patients to evaluate effectiveness and safety in ill people. In this phase, the researchers have to prove that the drug is a better treatment than any other currently available. It might be more effective; it might have fewer side effects; or it might be equivalent. These are usually large, double-blind, placebo-controlled studies. When these are done successfully, the results of all the studies are submitted to the FDA for review. Apart from certain "fast track" exceptions, this process takes at least two years. The FDA can approve the drug, reject it, or ask for further studies before they arrive at a conclusion. Once they approve a drug, it is monitored over the first few years of usage to see if further problems develop either in safety or effectiveness.

Doing these studies, as you can see, requires the participation of large numbers of volunteers. Should you be one of them? This is a difficult question that can in the end be answered only by the individual, but here are some of the pros and cons you might want to consider.

First the pros. If you participate in a clinical trial, you may get to try a new and effective treatment that is not otherwise available. You will get thorough (and free) health care during the course of the study. Some studies give extra compensation for travel or time spent in the study, although this varies depending on the study. Your participation is confidential, and you can withdraw from the treatment anytime you want. Finally, you are performing a service that may in the end help not only you, but thousands of other sufferers.

On the other hand, you're taking a chance: you may be getting a placebo—that is, no treatment at all for the course of the study—and neither you nor the researchers administering the treatment will know if you received a placebo until the study is finished. The time commitment can be considerable—these studies take as long as a year, and you will have to be available for frequent examinations over that time. You have to reveal complete information about your physical and mental health. Finally, medicines have side effects, and new medicines may have side effects no one knew about before the study began. Insurance companies may not pay for injury caused by an experimental drug.

There are a number of clinical trials going on right now, and of course more are starting regularly. At this writing there are clinical trials going on for treating chronic hepatitis B with recombinant beta interferon 1a, human anti–hepatitis B antibody, famciclovir, and lamivudine. For hepatitis C there are trials of beta interferon, beta 1a interferon, alpha 2a interferon, interferon alpha, consensus interferon, lymphoblastoid, thymosin, colony stimulating factor, and other drugs. These trials are being run at universities and drug companies, and some are in the later stages, almost ready for approval. The field is moving fast—so fast that a detailed list of the trials going on right now would be outdated by the time you read this. The best approach to finding what clinical trials are under way or getting under way is to check the Internet. A site called www.centerwatch.com, run by a Boston publishing company, lists (as of this writing) twenty-one different clinical trials in hepatitis treatments. It offers details on what is being studied, and gives addresses and telephone numbers. The sites are conveniently listed by state. The Liver Foundation (www.liverfoundation.org) also lists trials currently under way.

A Vaccine for Hepatitis C?

Hopes for the quick development of a vaccine after the discovery of the virus that causes hepatitis C have been dashed. For more than ten years researchers have worked to find an effective preventive, but progress has been extremely slow. With hepatitis A and B, the process was much easier—researchers knew that the body produced certain antibodies to these viruses, so duplicating their action in a vaccine was relatively simple. With hepatitis C it's another story. While some antibodies have been found, none of them produces immunity to subsequent infection, possibly because the hepatitis C virus changes its genetic makeup so readily and has so many different types and subtypes. Work on HCV vaccines goes on, but it has been proceeding for more than a decade without success. Still, some researchers are optimistic that within the next decade a vaccine or a treatment, or both, will be developed.

Basic Research

Spurred largely by the AIDS epidemic, there is a tremendous amount of basic research being done in the field of molecular virology. Much is now known about the genetic makeup of viruses and about how they replicate in the body. Interfering with or stopping the process of replication is the key to developing methods for slowing or eradicating the infection. Of course, this is an extremely complex process, and it happens at the cellular level—not an easy place to explore.

Researchers study the ways in which the hepatitis C virus forms proteins, and the steps by which new viruses are made and secreted out of the liver into the blood—the means by which the virus maintains the infection. Geneticists are examining how viral genes are copied to make new virus. The protease inhibitors that have been successful in treating AIDS are now being studied to see if there is one or more that will work for hepatitis C by inactivating the protease required for creating the molecules that form the viral particles. Some scientists are working on using frozen human liver cells as an infusion for people in liver failure. Others are working on cofactors in liver disease—abnormal bile salts (the enzyme that breaks down fat so that it can be digested), iron accumulation, the inflammatory properties of the cells, and so on. Working on drugs is only one approach: there is considerable work being done on the mechanisms of liver disease itself and how the damage done by the virus can be repaired even before there is an antiviral drug developed that will wipe out the virus.

But there are numerous, quite basic, unanswered questions. Why does hepatitis attack liver cells and not others? Why doesn't the liver cell destroy it as it would other invaders? What happens inside the cell to make it hospitable to the virus? We don't even fully understand the regenerative processes of the liver itself, or why fibrous tissue forms in cirrhosis. Answers to these and a thousand other questions are still to be discovered.

Afterword

Virology is such an active field of medical research that sometimes doctors will advise hepatitis patients who are relatively healthy, or for whom current treatments are inappropriate, to just live a healthy lifestyle and wait a while to see what develops. It is almost certain that pharmaceutical or genetic engineering companies, or government-sponsored researchers at university medical centers, will eventually develop a vaccine or a treatment for hepatitis C and a treatment for chronic hepatitis B. In fact, research in this area is proceeding so quickly that it was only as we were finishing this book that the Italian researchers discovered the S.E.N.-V virus.

That there are now safe and reliable vaccines for hepatitis A and hepatitis B does not mean that the threats posed by these diseases are ended. Having a vaccine and getting everyone vaccinated are two entirely different propositions. The vaccine for HBV has been in use now for more than fifteen years, but HBV is still a constant threat. Making HBV part of routine childhood vaccinations—and enforcing the procedure by denying unvaccinated kids admission to school—has helped. But it has not solved the problem. The CDC is confident that the vaccine is capable of wiping out HBV, if only it could be used widely enough. So far that has not happened.

Everyone waits eagerly for a vaccine for hepatitis C, the most disabling and deadly form of hepatitis. But in the meantime, the vaccines for hepatitis A and hepatitis B are not being effectively distributed and used. Creating a vaccine for hepatitis C is only the first step. Making it easily available and then convincing people to use it may prove almost as daunting a challenge.

For now, understanding your risk, and understanding how to minimize it, is the best approach. Seeking proper treatment from knowledgeable specialists is also essential, particularly in cases of hepatitis C. The disease is complex and extremely difficult to treat, and most physicians are not equipped to treat it effectively. You have to find those who are.

Appendix

Blood Tests and the Diagnosis of Liver Disease

There are some conditions or diseases where a blood test will tell you "whether you have it or you don't," but the tests for liver function don't fit this description. There are many tests that give some indication of how the liver is functioning, but, except for the tests that determine the presence of antibodies or actual viral load, they are not diagnostic of hepatitis. This does not mean that they are useless, but it does mean that they require expert interpretation by a physician who understands their meaning and limitations.

There are dozens of blood tests that are commonly performed, for example, when you get an annual physical. Among these might be tests for cholesterol and triglycerides, red blood cell count, potassium, white blood cell count, or platelet level, tests that give general information about bodily functions and health and, where substances are not at normal levels, may suggest to the doctor that further examination is required. Then there are tests performed to look for one specific factor—for example, tests to determine paternity, or those to detect illicit drug use. Next, there are many other tests that are only performed when the physician ordering the test has some special reason to do so. Most blood tests relevant to a patient who has or might have hepatitis fit into this group. They are informally called "liver function tests," and they may suggest many other things about the liver and other organs in addition to damage from hepatitis. Their results are not self-evident, and not always subject to easy interpretation, even by experienced physicians. And finally, there are many tests whose clinical significance is unknown or not firmly established but which are performed as components of research protocols.

Among the many complications of liver function tests is that on the one hand they can be normal in people who nevertheless have chronic hepatitis, and on the other can indicate problems that have little to do with the functioning of the liver itself but may suggest malfunctions in other organs. A given blood test alone, without a full clinical picture of your health, will tell the doctor little about how to proceed.

The following is a listing of the most common blood tests run for suspected or actual hepatitis infections, along with a brief discussion of their meaning.

ALT (alanine aminotransferase). Normal values: 5–35 international units/liter. Values on this test may increase because of hepatitis, cirrhosis, liver tumor, drugs that are poisonous to the liver, or cholestasis (a slowing or stopping of bile flow). Mildly elevated levels of ALT may be normal for gender, certain ethnic groups, or body mass index. Men, blacks, and Hispanics tend to have higher ALT values, as do obese people whose livers are fatty. ALT level correlates only moderately well with liver inflammation in chronic liver diseases such as hepatitis C—in fact, almost one-third of hepatitis C patients have normal ALT levels. Still, ALT levels are higher in those with liver inflammation than in those without. ALT levels can increase after a muscle injury, including the injury to the heart muscle during a heart attack, or even in response to severe muscle exertion.

AST (aspartate aminotransferase). Normal values: 5–40 international units/liter. Increased values here may indicate hepatitis, cirrhosis, acute pancreatitis, skeletal muscle trauma, liver tumor, or any of a number of different muscle diseases. Readings may be lower in pregnant women and in people with diabetic ketoacidosis (excessive amounts of ketones in the blood and urine of diabetics).

AP (alkaline phosphatase). Normal values: 30–85 international units/liter. AP is found in the liver, the biliary system, bone, intestines, and white blood cells. Levels can be elevated in a number of disorders that affect the drainage of bile—for example, gallstones or a tumor blocking the common bile duct. Alcoholic liver disease, cirrhosis, or a liver tumor can also cause increased levels, as can rheumatoid arthritis and other bone diseases. (The test can also determine how much of the AP comes from the liver and how much from the bone.) Low levels can indicate protein or vitamin deficiency as well as other kinds of malnutrition.

GGT (gamma-glutamyl transpeptidase). Normal values: 5–38 international units/liter. This enzyme is mainly found in liver cells, and as liver cells die, it leaks out into the blood. Levels are elevated in liver disorders, but, unlike alkaline phosphatase, not elevated in diseases of the bone. Elevated levels are found in alcoholism, bile duct obstruction, and drug abuse. The aftermath of a heart attack can also produce elevated levels of GGT.

Bilirubin. Normal values: 0.1–1 mg/dl (total); 0.1–0.3 mg/dl (conjugated); 0.2–0.8 mg/dl (unconjugated). Bilirubin is a waste product produced when red blood cells die due to damage or aging. The liver removes the substance from the blood, and to the extent it fails to do so it isn't functioning properly. So excess amounts of bilirubin in the blood indicate that the liver isn't doing its job. Normally there is only a small amount of bilirubin circulating in the blood; excess amounts cause jaundice, the yellowish tint of the skin and eyes typical of liver malfunction. Elevated bilirubin is nonspecific—it can indicate many different forms of liver or biliary tract disease—but it is a true test of liver function because it reflects how well the liver is performing one of its many essential functions. Bilirubin levels cannot, however, be used to determine the severity of hepatitis. "Unconjugated" bilirubin is formed from biliverdin, the excretory product of hemoglobin, and is fat soluble. It binds to albumin before being transported to the liver. The liver converts it into "conjugated" bilirubin, a water-soluble form that can be excreted. Elevation of the conjugated bilirubin level may suggest that the liver is all right but the bile duct isn't functioning properly. Elevation of unconjugated bilirubin may mean the liver itself isn't doing the job of converting the substance into its conjugated form.

Serum albumin. Normal values: 3.2–5 g/dl. Albumin is a protein manufactured by the liver and found in the blood. Decreased levels of it occur in malnutrition, diarrhea, fever, infection, inadequate iron intake, and in lupus, Crohn's disease, and liver disease, among other illnesses. The test, in other words, is nonspecific, but if other diseases are ruled out, low albumin levels suggest a poor prognosis for someone with liver disease.

Prothrombin time. Normal values: 11 to 12.5 seconds. This is a test of blood clotting. All blood clotting factors except Factor VIII are synthesized by the liver, and failure of blood to clot quickly enough is an indication that the liver is not functioning properly. There is a high degree of correlation between extended times on this test and the degree of liver damage. Usually by the time this test is abnormal, liver disease is fairly advanced. Prothrombin time can be prolonged in cases of vitamin K deficiency, by certain drugs (anticoagulants, for example), and some non-liver disorders.

Platelet count. Normal values: 130,000–400,000. Decreased levels of platelets may indicate an immune system failure, and are characteristic of a number of serious conditions, including bone marrow diseases. Platelets are also essential to proper blood coagulation.

Serum ammonia. Normal values: less than 50 mg/dl. Ammonia, a water-soluble gas, is formed in the body as it metabolizes protein. The liver converts it into urea so that it can be excreted by the kidneys. Elevated levels of ammonia may suggest liver malfunction, but even patients with advanced liver disease can have normal readings. Ammonia levels correlate with encephalopathy (brain disease), which is one of the potentially fatal complications of liver disease.

A/G ratio (albumin/globulin ratio). Normal values: 0.8–2. This is a calculated value arrived at by dividing the albumin level by the globulin level. Lower levels may suggest liver malfunction, kidney malfunction, or infection, but higher readings are not clinically significant.

BUN (blood urea nitrogen). Normal values: 7–25 mg/dl. Urea is the main end product of protein metabolism that the liver produces for excretion in urine. If levels are too high, this may mean that the kidneys are not functioning properly; if they are too low, then the problem may be in the liver. Decreased BUN levels can also be caused by poor diet.

Blood Tests for the Presence of HCV

ELISA (enzyme linked immunosorbent assay). This test detects biochemical sequences that correspond to the antibodies in the hepatitis C virus. Antibodies show only exposure to the virus, not the presence of the virus itself. Antibodies are not formed for as much as six months after exposure, so the test is of limited usefulness although it is inexpensive and often used as a screening test for HCV. Both false positives and false negatives, however, are common.

RIBA (recombinant immunoblot assay). This test is more reliable than the ELISA in determining HCV infection. It detects biochemical patterns that correspond to HCV antibodies. The test is fairly reliable, but it has to be interpreted by a pathologist by comparing the result to a control sample. It is more expensive than the ELISA, and is commonly given after a positive ELISA as a means of confirming the diagnosis, particularly in low-risk populations.

HCV RNA by PCR (polymerase chain reaction). This is the most sensitive of the HCV tests. It tests for the presence of the virus itself, not its antibodies, and can detect HCV in blood and other tissues. The test takes a sample of the blood and then amplifies the virus's nucleic acid—a chain reaction that results in millions of copies of the nucleic acid, which can then be detected. It can also tell how much virus was present in the original sample. It can detect the virus as soon as three days after infection. Some genotypes of the virus are more easily detected than others. Different laboratories have different ways of reporting the results, and comparisons can be difficult. A negative result on this test does not necessarily mean that the virus has cleared. It may still be present in undetectable amounts. PCR is the most sensitive test, but it is prone to false positives, and is not approved for diagnosis.

B-DNA for HCV. Another test for the presence of the virus itself, but somewhat less sensitive than the PCR.

Genotype tests. These are the tests that determine what genotype of the hepatitis C virus is causing the infection. Such tests will not usually affect the treatment you receive, but may be useful in predicting the efficacy of such treatment under certain circumstances. They are at this time more useful in research than in clinical practice.

Resources

Organizations and Support Groups

American Association for the Study of Liver Diseases
    (AASLD)
6900 Grove Rd.
Thorofare, NJ 08086
(609) 848–1000
www.hepar-sfgh.ucsf.edu

American College of Gastroenterology
4900 B South 31st St.
Arlington, VA 22206
(703) 820–7400
fax: (703) 931–4520
www.acg.gi.org

American Liver Foundation
1425 Pompton Ave.
Cedar Grove, NJ 07009
(800) 465–4837 or (888) 443–7222
www.liverfoundation.org

Centers for Disease Control and Prevention (CDC)
Hepatitis Branch; Mailstop G37
1600 Clifton Rd. NE
Atlanta, GA 30333
CDC Hepatitis Hotline:
    (888) 443–7232
www.cdc.gov/ncidod/diseases/hepatitis/hepatitis.htm

Digestive Health Initiative
7910 Woodmont Ave., Suite 700
Bethesda, MD 20814
(800) 668–5237
www.gastro.org/dhi.html

European Association for the Study of the Liver (EASL)
EASL Liaison Bureau
Hepatology Unit—Hôpital Necker
149, rue de Sèvres
75747 Paris, Cedex 15
France
fax: 33 1 44 49 51 65
e-mail: isabelle.porteret@nck.ap-hop-paris.fr

Hepatitis B Foundation
700 East Butler Ave.
Doylestown, PA 18901–2697
(215) 489–4900
www2.hepb.org/hepb/
e-mail: info@hepb.org

Hepatitis C Foundation
1502 Russett Dr.
Warminster, PA 18972
(215) 672–2606
fax: (215) 672–1518
www.hepcfoundation.org

Hepatitis Foundation International
30 Sunrise Terrace
Cedar Grove, NJ 07009–1423
(800) 891–0707
www.hepfi.org
e-mail: hfi@intac.com

HCV Global Foundation
2807 Swan Way
Fairfield, CA 94533
(707) 425–5343
fax: (510) 569–3743
e-mail: vironn@aol.com

Hep-C ALERT, Inc.
2630 Hollywood Blvd., Suite 100
Hollywood, FL 33020
(954) 920-5277
toll-free: 877-HELP-4-HEP (877–435–7443)
fax: (954) 920–7577
www.hep-C-alert.org

Hepatitis Education Project
P.O. Box 95162
Seattle, WA 98145
e-mail: graham@phoenix.artsci.washington.edu

Immunization Action Coalition (IAC)/The Hepatitis B
    Coalition
1573 Selby Ave., Suite 234
St Paul, MN 55104
www.immunize.org

National Digestive Diseases Information Clearinghouse
2 Information Way
Bethesda, MD 20892–3570
(301) 654–3810
www.niddk.nih.gov

National Foundation for Infectious Diseases (NFID)
4733 Bethesda Ave., Suite 750
Bethesda, MD 20814
(301) 656–0003
www.medscape.com/Affiliates/NFID/

National Institute of Diabetes and Digestive and Kidney
    Diseases (NIDDK)
2 Information Way
Bethesda, MD 20892–3570
(301) 654–3810
www.niddk.nih.gov

National Institutes of Health
Two divisions of this federal government agency conduct
    research on hepatitis: the National Institute of Allergy
    and Infectious Diseases (NIAAID), and the National
    Institute of Diabetes and Digestive and Kidney
    Diseases (NIDDK)
NIAID Office of Communication
Building 31, Room 7A50
Bethesda, MD 20892
(301) 496–5717
www.niddk.niaid.gov/index.htm

United Liver Association
11646 West Pico Blvd.
Los Angeles, CA 90064
(310) 914–8252

Periodicals

Hepatitis Weekly
C.W. Henderson Publications
www.newsfile.com/11.htm

Focus: On Hepatitis
Quantum Media Group
130 Prim Road
Colchester, VT 05446
(802) 655–2715

Hep-C Connection
1714 Poplar Street
Denver, CO 80220
(303) 393–9395

Bibliography

Books

Askari, Fred K. *Hepatitis C: The Silent Epidemic*. New York: Plenum, 1999.

Dolan, Matthew. *The Hepatitis C Handbook*. Berkeley, Calif.: North Atlantic, 1999.

Everson, Gregory, and Hedy Weinberg. *Living with Hepatitis C: A Survivor's Guide*. New York: Hatherleigh, 1998.

Roybal, Beth Ann Petro. *Hepatitis C: A Personal Guide to Good Health*. Berkeley, Calif.: Ulysses, 1997.

Specter, Steven. *Viral Hepatitis: Diagnosis, Therapy, and Prevention*. Totowa, N.J.: Humana, 1999.

Turkington, Carol. *Hepatitis C: The Silent Killer*. Chicago: Contemporary Books, 1998.

Scientific Papers

General Papers on Viral Hepatitis

Centers for Disease Control and Prevention. "Protection against viral hepatitis: Recommendations of the immunization practices advisory committee (ACIP)." *MMWR* 39 (No. RR-2) (1990): 1–26.

Koff, R. S. "Advances in the treatment of chronic viral hepatitis." *Journal of the American Medical Association* 282:6 (Aug. 1999): 511–12.

Loscher, T., J. S. Keystone, and R. Steffen. "Vaccination of travelers against hepatitis A and B." *Journal of Travel Medicine* 6:2 (1999): 107–14.

Hepatitis A

Centers for Disease Control and Prevention. "Prevention of hepatitis A through active or passive immunization: recommendations of the advisory committee on immunization practices (ACIP)." *MMWR* 48 (No. RR-12) (1999): 48.

———. "Hepatitis A vaccination of men who have sex with men—Atlanta, Georgia, 1996–1997." *MMWR* 47:34 (1998): 708–11.

———. "Hepatitis A vaccination programs in communities with high rates of hepatitis A." *MMWR* 46:28 (1997): 600–603.

———. "Notice of readers licensure of inactivated hepatitis A vaccine and recommendations for use among international travelers." *MMWR* 44:29 (1995): 559–60.

———. "Foodborne hepatitis A—Missouri, Wisconsin, and Alaska, 1990–1992." *MMWR* 42:27 (1993): 526–29.

Doebbeling, B. N., N. Li, and R. P. Wenzel. "An outbreak of hepatitis A among health care workers: risk factors for transmission." *American Journal of Public Health* 83 (1993): 1679–84.

Hadler, S. C., and L. McFarlane. "Hepatitis in day care centers: epidemiology and prevention." *Review of Infectious Diseases* 8 (1986): 548–57.

Katz, M. H., L. Hsu, E. Wong, et al. "Seroprevalence of and risk factors for hepatitis A infection among young homosexual and bisexual men." *Journal of Infectious Disease* 175 (1997): 1225–29.

Niu, M. T., L. B. Polish, J. D. Smith, et al. "Multistate outbreak of hepatitis A associated with frozen strawberries." *Journal of Infectious Disease* 166 (1992): 518–24.

Pickering, L. K. "Infections in day care." *Pediatric Infectious Diseases* 6 (1987): 614–17.

Reves, R. R., and L. K. Pickering. "Impact of child day care on infectious diseases in adults." *Infectious Disease Clinics of North America* 6 (1992): 239–50.

Winokur, P. L., and J. R. Stapleton. "Immunoglobulin prophylaxis for hepatitis A." *Clin. Infect. Dis.* 14 (1992): 580–86.

Hepatitis B

Centers for Disease Control and Prevention. "Update: Recommendations to prevent hepatitis B virus transmission—United States." *MMWR* 48:2 (1999): 33–34.

———. "Hepatitis B virus: A comprehensive strategy for eliminating transmission in the United States through universal childhood vaccination: Recommendations of the immunization practices advisory committee (ACIP)." *MMWR* 40 (No. RR-13) (1991): 1–19.

———. "Public health service inter-agency guidelines for screening donors of blood, plasma, organs, tissues, and semen for evidence of hepatitis B and C." *MMWR* 40 (No. RR-4) (1991): 1–17.

Niederau et al. "Long-term follow-up of HBeAg-positive patients treated with interferon alfa for chronic hepatitis B." *New England Journal of Medicine* 334 (1998): 1422–27.

Perrillo, R., J. Rakela, P. Martin, et al. "Lamivudine Transplant Study Group. Lamivudine for hepatitis B after liver transplantation." *Hepatology* 24 (1996): 182a.

Wright, T. L. and J. Y. N. Lau. "Clinical aspects of hepatitis B virus infection." *Lancet* 342 (1993): 1340–44.

Hepatitis C

Bonkovsky et al. "Reduction of health-related quality of life in chronic hepatitis C and improvement with interferon therapy." *Hepatology* 29 (1999): 264–70.

Centers for Disease Control and Prevention. "Recommendations for prevention and control of hepatitis C virus (HCV) infection and HCV-related chronic disease." *MMWR* 47 (No. RR-19) (1998).

———. "Transmission of hepatitis C virus infection associated with home infusion therapy for hemophilia." *MMWR* 46:28 (1997): 597–99.

———. "Recommendations for follow-up of healthcare workers after occupational exposure to hepatitis C virus." *MMWR* 46:28 (1997): 603–6.

Di Bisceglie, A. M., and B. R. Bacon. "The Unmet Challenges of Hepatitis C." *Scientific American*, October 1999, 80–85.

Foster, G. R., R. D. Goldin, and H. C. Thomas. "Chronic hepatitis C infection causes a significant reduction in quality of life in the absence of cirrhosis." *Hepatology* 27:1 (Jan. 1998): 209–12.

Kubo, S., S. Nishiguchi, et al. "Clinical significance of prior hepatitis B virus infection in patients with hepatitis C virus–related hepatocellular carcinoma." *Cancer* 86:5 (Sept. 1, 1999): 793–98.

McHutchinson, J. G., et al. "Interferon Alfa 2b alone or in combination with ribavirin as initial treatment for chronic hepatitis C." *New England Journal of Medicine* 339:21 (Nov. 19, 1999): 1485–92.

Reddy, K. R., J. H. Hoofnagle, et al. "Racial differences in responses to therapy with interferon in chronic hepatitis C." Consensus Interferon Study Group. *Hepatology* 30:3 (Sept. 1999): 787–93.

Shehab, T. M., S. S. Sonnad, M. Jeffries, N. Gunaratnum, and A. S. Lok. "Current practice patterns of primary care physicians in the management of patients with hepatitis C." *Hepatology* 30:30 (Sept. 1999): 794–800.

Wietzke, P., P. Schott, F. Braun, S. Mihm, and G. Ramadori. "Clearance of HCV RNA in chronic hepatitis C virus–infected patients during acute hepatitis B virus superinfection." *Liver* 19:4 (Aug. 1999): 348–53.

You, S., M. Zhou, et al. "A clinical study on bing gan ling oral liquid for treatment of hepatitis C." *Journal of Traditional Chinese Medicine* 18:3 (Sept. 1998): 209–14.

Hepatitis D

Battegay, M., L. H. Simpson, et al. "Elimination of hepatitis delta virus infection after loss of hepatitis B surface antigen in patients with chronic delta hepatitis." *Journal of Medical Virology* 44:4 (Dec. 1994): 389–92.

Bichko, V., H. J. Netter, T. T. Wu, et al. "Pathogenesis associated with replication of hepatitis delta virus." *Infect Agents Dis* 3:2–3 (Apr.–June 1994): 94–97.

Casey, J. L. "Hepatitis delta virus. Genetics and pathogenesis." *Clinical Laboratory Medicine* 16:2 (June 1996): 451–64.

Chen, P. J., H. L. Wu, C. J. Wang, et al. "Molecular biology of hepatitis D virus: research and potential for application." *Journal of Gastroenterological Hepatology* 12:9–10 (Oct. 1997): S188–92.

Eyster, M. E., J. C. Sanders, M. Beggegay, and A. M. Di Bisceglie. "Suppression of hepatitis C virus (HCV) replication by hepatitis D virus (HDV) in HIV-infected hemophiliacs with chronic hepatitis B and C." *Dig Dis Sci* 40:7 (July 1995): 1583–88.

Farci, P., P. Karayiannis, M. G. Brook, et al. "Treatment of chronic hepatitis delta virus (HDV) infection with human lymphoblastoid alpha interferon." *Q J Med* 73:271 (Nov. 1989): 1045–54.

Farci, P., P. Karayiannis, M. E. Lai, et al. "Acute and chronic hepatitis delta virus infection: direct or indirect effect on hepatitis B virus replication?" *Journal of Medical Virology* 26:3 (Nov. 1988): 279–88.

Gerken, G., and K. H. Meyer zum Buschenfelde. "Chronic hepatitis delta virus (HDV) infection." *Hepatogastroenterology* 38:1 (Feb. 1999): 29–32.

Hadziyannis, S. J. "Review: hepatitis delta." *Journal of Gastroenterological Hepatology* 12:4 (Apr. 1997): 280–98.

Ichimura, H., I. Tamura, T. Tsubakio, O. Kurimura, and T. Kurimura. "Influence of hepatitis delta virus superinfection on the clearance of hepatitis B virus (HBV) markers in HBV carriers in Japan." *Journal of Medical Virology* 26:1 (Sept. 1988): 49–55.

Karayiannis, P. "Hepatitis D virus." *Review of Medical Virology* 8:1 (Jan. 1998): 13–24.

Karayiannis, P., J. Saldanha, J. Monjardino, P. Farci, and H. C. Thomas. "Prevention and treatment of hepatitis delta virus infection." *Prog. Clin Biol Res* 364 (1991): 377–83.

Krogsgaard, K., P. Wantzin, L. Mathiesen, et al. "Chronic evolution of acute hepatitis B: the significance of simultaneous infections with hepatitis C and D." Copenhagen Hepatitis Acuta Programme. Scan J; *Gastroenterology* 26:3 (March 1991): 275–80.

Lai, M. M. "The molecular biology of hepatitis delta virus." *Annual Review of Biochemistry* 64 (1995): 259–86.

Lau, D. T., Y. Doo E Park, D. E. Kleiner, P. Schmid, M. C. Kuhns, and J. H. Hoofnagle. "Lamivudine for chronic delta hepatitis." *Hepatology* 30:2 (Aug. 1999): 546–49.

Makino, S., M. F. Chang, C. K. Shieh, et al. "Molecular cloning and sequencing of a human hepatitis delta (delta) virus RNA." *Nature* 329:6137 (Sept. 24–30, 1987): 343–46.

Monjardino, J. "Replication of hepatitis delta virus." *Journal of Viral Hepatology* 3:4 (July 1996): 163–66.

Monjardino, J. P., and J. A. Saldanha. "Delta hepatitis. The disease and the virus." *British Medical Bulletin* 46:2 (Apr. 1990): 399–407.

Niro, G. A., J. L. Casey, et al. "Intrafamilial transmission of hepatitis D virus: molecular evidence." *Journal of Hepatology* 30:4 (Apr. 1999): 564–69.

Poss, J. E. "Hepatitis D virus infection." *Nurse Practitioner* 14:8 (Aug. 1989): 12, 14–15, 18.

Rizzetto, M. "Hepatitis delta virus (HDV) infection and disease." *Ric Clin Lab* 19:1 (Jan.–Mar. 1989): 11–26.

Rizzetto, M., A. Ponzetto, and I. Forzani. "Hepatitis delta virus as a global health problem." *Vaccine* 8 Suppl. (Mar. 1990): S10–14; discussion S21–23.

Rosina, F., P. Conoscitore, R. Cuppone, et al. "Changing pattern of chronic hepatitis D in Southern Europe." *Gastroenterology* 117:1 (July 1999): 161–66.

Sakugawa, H., H. Nakasone, et al. "Determination of hepatitis delta virus (HDV)-RNA in asymptomatic cases of HDV infection." *American Journal of Gastroenterology* 92:12 (Dec. 1997): 2232–36.

Hepatitis E

Clayson, E. T., D. W. Vaugn, B. L. Innis, et al. "Association of hepatitis E virus with an outbreak of hepatitis at a military training camp in Nepal." *Journal of Medical Virology* 54:3 (March 1998): 178–82.

Coursaget, P., Y. Buisson, M. N. N'gawara, et al. "Outbreak of enterically-transmitted hepatitis due to hepatitis A and hepatitis E viruses." *Journal of Hepatology* 28:5 (May 1998): 745–50.

———. "Role of hepatitis E virus in sporadic cases of acute and fulminant hepatitis in an endemic area (Chad)." *Am J Trop Med Hyg* 58:3 (March 1998): 330–34.

Coursaget, P., D. Krawczynski, Y. Buisson, et al. "Hepatitis E and hepatitis C virus infections among French soldiers with non-A, non-B hepatitis." *Journal of Medical Virology* 39:2 (Feb. 1993): 163–66.

Mast, E., J. Alter, P. V. Holland, et al. "Evaluation of assays for antibody to hepatitis E virus by a serum panel." *Hepatology* 27:3 (March 1998): 857–61.

Tsega, E., K. Krawczynski, B. G. Hansson, et al. "Outbreak of acute hepatitis E virus infection among military personnel in northern Ethiopia." *Journal of Medical Virology* 34:4 (Aug. 1991): 232–36.

Hepatitis G

Di Bisceglie, A. M. "Hepatitis G virus infection: a work in progress." *Annals of Internal Medicine* 125 (Nov. 1996): 772–73.

Tanaka, E., Y. Nakatsuji, M. Kobayashi, et al. "Two patients with acute hepatitis B with suspected sexual transmission of hepatitis G virus." *Journal of Gastroenterology* 33:3 (June 1998): 419–23.

Tanaka, E., M. Tacke, M. Kobayashi, et al. "Past and present hepatitis G infections in areas where hepatitis C is highly endemic and those where it is not endemic." *Journal of Clinical Microbiology* 36:1 (Jan. 1998): 110–14.

Tanaka, T., G. Hess, S. Tanaka, et al. "The significance of hepatitis G virus infection in patients with non-A to C hepatic diseases." *Hepatogastroenterology* 46:27 (May–June 1999): 1870–73.

Index

Page numbers of charts or graphs appear in italics.